5 minute first aid

Tear out this card and keep it with you at all times – you never know when you may need it.

British Red Cross
Caring for people in crisis

Bleeding

To control severe bleeding:

- Press on the wound (over clean material, if at hand).
- Elevate the wound above the level of the heart.
- Apply a dressing.
- Treat for shock, reassure and keep warm, lay the person down, raise the feet, loosen tight clothing.

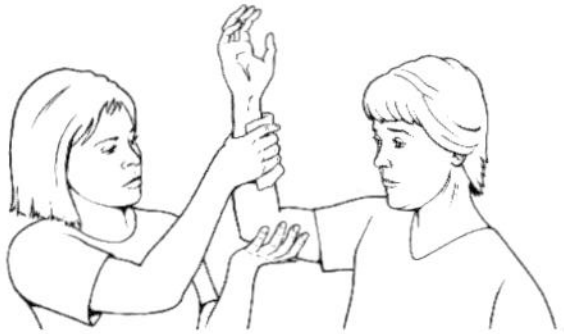

General advice

- Reassure the person and keep them warm.
- Do not move the person unnecessarily.
- Do not give cigarettes or anything to eat or drink.

If in doubt, call an ambulance.

British Red Cross
For more information about our training courses, first aid supplies and all our first aid learning products – call: 0870 170 9222
visit: www.redcross.org.uk/firstaid
email: firstaid@redcross.org.uk

British Red Cross
Caring for people in crisis

5 minute first aid

first aid essentials

In the event of an emergency, it's vital that you stop, get involved and keep calm. Follow these simple steps:

Assess the injured person

- Danger – are you or the person in danger?
- Response – is the person conscious?
- Airway – is the airway o
- Breathing – is the persc

Act on your findings

Person conscious, bre

- Treat any injuries.

Person unconscious, b

- Treat any life-threatening
- Place in the recovery pc

Recovery position

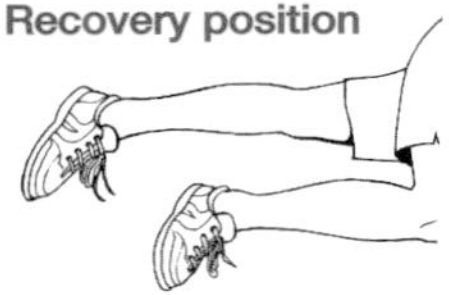

GW00361788

Opening the airway

- Look in the mouth and remove obvious obstructions. Tilt the head and lift the chin.
- Look, listen and feel for breathing.

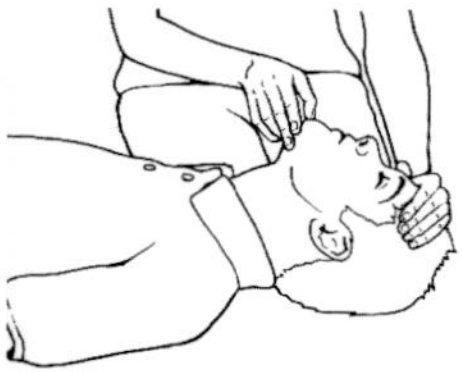

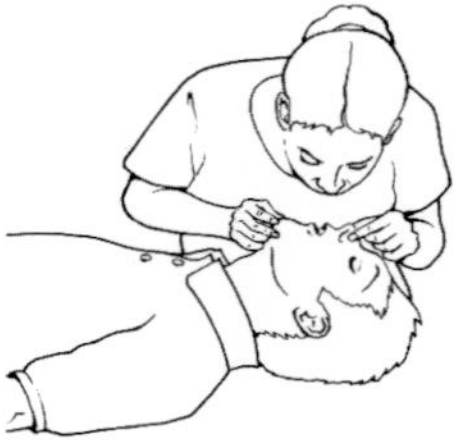

Person unconscious**, breathing** absent

- Send a helper to call 999.
- Give 2 rescue breaths.
- Assess circulation by checking for signs of life.

Breathing for the person

- Ensure good seals at:
  a the nostrils (with finger/thumb);
  b the mouth (with your mouth).
- Blow into the person's lungs until chest rises.
- Remove lips. Allow chest to fall. After every 10 breaths (about 1 minute), re-check for signs of circulation.

Person unconscious**, breathing** absent **and circulation present**

- Continue rescue breaths.
- Re-check for circulation every minute.

Person unconscious**, breathing** absent **and circulation** absent

- Combine rescue breaths with chest compressions.
- Repeat until help arrives.

Giving chest compressions

If chest compressions are required:

- Find the lower half of the breastbone.
- Compress the chest to a depth of 4–5 cms at a rate of 100 per minute.
- After every 15 compressions, give 2 breaths.
- Continue until help arrives or the person starts to breathe again.

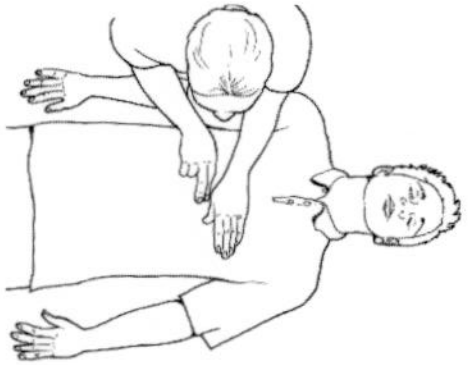

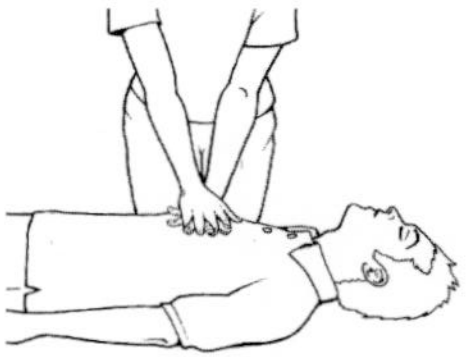

Remember DR ABC – **Danger**, **Response**, **Airway**, **Breathing**, **Circulation**.

British Red Cross

Caring for people in crisis

5 minute first aid

for travel

Hodder Arnold

A MEMBER OF THE HODDER HEADLINE GROUP

Orders: Please contact Bookpoint Ltd, 130 Milton Park, Abingdon, Oxon OX14 4SB. Telephone: (44) 01235 827720, Fax: (44) 01235 400454. Lines are open from 9.00 to 18.00, Monday to Saturday, with a 24-hour message answering service. You can also order through our website www.hoddereducation.com

British Library Cataloguing in Publication Data
A catalogue record for this title is available from the British Library.

ISBN-10: 0 340 90465 8
ISBN-13: 9 780340 904657

First published	2005
Impression number	10 9 8 7 6 5 4 3 2 1
Year	2008 2007 2006 2005

Typeset by Transet Limited, Coventry, England.
Printed in Great Britain for Hodder Arnold, a division of Hodder Headline, 338 Euston Road, London NW1 3BH, by Cox & Wyman Ltd, Reading, Berkshire.

Hodder Headline's policy is to use papers that are natural, renewable and recyclable products and made from wood grown in sustainable forests. The logging and manufacturing processes are expected to conform to the environmental regulations of the country of origin.

contents

acknowledgements

The authors would like to pay special thanks to Charlotte Hall, Catherine Jones, Genevieve Okech, Naomi Safir and Roger Smith.

preface

The British Red Cross, as part of the International Red Cross and Red Crescent Movement, is the world's largest first-aid training organization. With over 180 Red Cross societies worldwide we endeavour to make first-aid knowledge and skills accessible to individuals, families, schools and the wider community.

You never know when someone may need your help but it is highly likely that when called on to provide emergency first aid it will be to someone close to you such as a friend or a member of your own family. Therefore, we have produced the *Five-minute First Aid* series in order to give you the relevant skills and confidence needed to be able to save a life and help an injured person, whatever your situation.

We appreciate that it is difficult to find time in hectic lifestyles to learn first-aid skills. Consequently, this series is designed so that you can learn and absorb each specific, essential skill that is relevant to you in just five minutes and you can pick up and put down the book as you wish. The features throughout the book will help you to reinforce what you have learnt and will build your confidence in applying first aid.

5 • 5

This book is divided into five-minute sections, so that you can discover each invaluable skill in just a short amount of time.

one-minute wonder

One-minute wonders ask and answer the questions that you might be thinking as you read.

key skills

The key skill features emphasize and reiterate the main skills of the section – helping you to commit them to memory and recall them when necessary.

summary

Summary sections summarize the key points of the chapter in order to further consolidate your knowledge and understanding.

self-testers

The self-testers ensure that you have learnt the most important facts of the chapter. They will give you an indication of how much you are absorbing as you go along and help to build your confidence. (Note: some of the multiple choice questions may have more than one possible answer!)

We hope that this book will give you the opportunity to learn the most important skills you will ever need in a friendly, straightforward way and that it prepares you for any first-aid situation that you may encounter.

introduction

Accidents will happen, whether you are at home or abroad, and we know that thousands of people receive injuries or become unwell each year while travelling or on holiday. Some of these people could be helped if the first person on the scene had known first aid and was prepared to get involved.

In this book, we highlight the things you can do to make a difference; we describe the first-aid care in an easy-to-understand language, and we are sensitive to the challenges facing you as a potential first aider.

It is important to remember that in extreme cases first aid can be the difference between life and death. On other occasions, it can stop the person's condition from becoming worse and, in some cases, there may be an improvement in the person. However, all of this depends on you having the appropriate skills and knowledge, and being prepared to do something if you come across a situation requiring first aid.

We appreciate that going on holiday is a time of anticipation and excitement, and being involved in an accident or becoming unwell is probably the last thing on your mind. There is no way to predict when a car accident will happen or when the person on the beach will have a heart attack. Yet all the evidence tells us that it will happen and, when it does, the person needing your care will be known to you; the odds are that it will be a member of your family. So be prepared, learn the first-aid skills that will make a difference and take this knowledge with you on every journey you make.

For convenience and clarity, we use the pronoun 'he' when referring to the first aider and injured person.

1

how to deal with an emergency

It is difficult to think about the possibility of an unexpected emergency when travelling, especially if you are excited about going on holiday or visiting friends. Nevertheless, by its very nature an emergency is unexpected and it is important to know what to do. Travel can range from undertaking a solitary activity such as walking in the hills, to waiting for a flight in a crowded airport; the main consideration for dealing with an unexpected emergency is the facility to call for help. The increased availability of mobile telephones and the ability to pinpoint a person's whereabouts using global positioning systems (GPS) make calling for help much easier than it used to be, and everyone should know how to call for help in an emergency. A simple measure such as telling someone where you are going may be life saving.

an emergency situation

When you find yourself dealing with an unexpected emergency, it is important to make sure that you are not putting yourself in danger. If there is obvious danger, call the emergency services and wait for them to arrive before approaching the incident. It is also important to keep bystanders away from the danger – warn them if you can. There is a range of things that may pose a risk to you when dealing with an emergency situation and some of the more common dangers are listed on pages 4 and 5. However, the ultimate decision rests with you at the time, but remember you will not be in a position to help anyone if you end up as a casualty yourself. It is also important to keep bystanders away from the danger, so warn them if you can. We in the British Red Cross have been delivering first aid for more than 100 years. We know that first-aid incidents in public places attract a large number of onlookers, many of whom are prepared to get involved and help. Some of these situations are poorly handled because no one has stepped forward and demonstrated any leadership qualities, assessed the danger, delegated responsibility or started to deliver immediate care.

calling for help

Everyone, when faced with an emergency, feels some anxiety. Consequently, it is a good idea to shout loudly to see if anyone can come to help you. You will feel less anxious if you have someone else with you, and another person can help if you are faced with several tasks at once, such as:

- securing and maintaining the safety of the scene
- calling for the emergency services
- bringing first-aid equipment
- maintaining a person's privacy
- helping with first aid, especially if there is more than one injured person.

All bystanders can be helpful if they are given clear instructions and if they are kept busy. Try and act with authority and give helpers clear orders. This may reduce the panic and confusion that always surrounds a significant emergency. If you are the most experienced first aider present, take control and tell others you are trained to give first aid. If other first aiders come forward, ask them to help to locate and assess the injured people. Try to keep a clear picture of what is happening so that you can pass on accurate information to the emergency services. If you do ask a bystander to call the emergency services, make sure this is done.

calling the emergency services

To call the emergency services in the UK, you must dial 999; in the European Union (EU), dial 112. The emergency number will be different in countries outside the EU – it is a good idea to know the number in the country you are visiting.

In the UK, it is possible to contact the fire, police, ambulance, mountain rescue, fell rescue, cave rescue, mine rescue and coastguard services using 999. When you dial 999, you will be asked which service you need. If it is a significant emergency with several people involved or, if safety is a problem, you will need fire, police and ambulance.

The operator will ask you for some information about the emergency, and so it is important to know some answers before you phone, such as your location and your phone number. You will also be asked to give an indication of the type and seriousness of the emergency, the number of injured people and whether or not there are any dangers such as chemicals or toxic fumes.

be aware of the dangers

Examples of danger that would prevent you from approaching the scene include:

- smoke, fire and flames
- toxic fumes/hazardous chemicals (see Figure 1)
- bomb blast
- flying bullets
- falling masonry
- high voltage electricity

- swirling or deep water or flood water (especially if you are a non-swimmer)
- iced-over ponds.

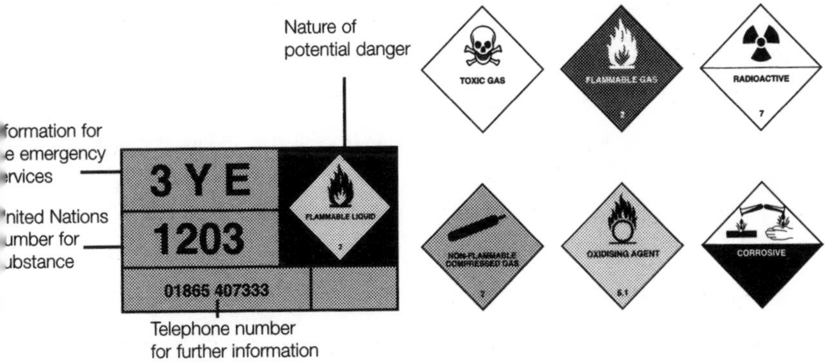

Fig 1 The HAZCHEM card
In the event of a road traffic accident vehicles carrying hazardous chemicals will carry the HAZCHEM card.

If there is no serious danger and you think it is safe to approach an incident, try to find out what has happened and how many people are involved. Remember that some may have left the scene or been thrown from a moving vehicle.

specific incidents

car crash

If you come across a car crash and it is safe to approach, park your vehicle safely, switch on your hazard lights, and alert the emergency services. At a car crash site you will usually need police, fire and ambulance services. Use your warning triangles.

(It is breaking the law to travel without warning triangles in some parts of Europe). Place them on the side of the road where other drivers can see them as they approach. The triangles should be at least 45 m away from the crash in either direction. Send bystanders to warn other drivers. Stabilize any vehicles involved in the crash by switching off the ignition and applying the handbrake. Make sure you look for all the injured people.

one-minute wonder

Q If I am treating a person in the middle of the road, should I move him first?

A It is important that you do not move the person until you have assessed his injuries (see page 10). If you suspect a back or neck injury, you must not move him at all. Instead ask bystanders to stop the traffic.

fire

If you are staying in a hotel or hostel, always take time to familiarize yourself with what to do in case of a fire, and make sure you know where the fire exits are.

If you are aware of a fire or of smoke, sound the fire alarm and warn as many people as possible in the area of the fire. Remember that fire and smoke can spread quickly.

If the fire alarm sounds, it is essential to think quickly in order to evacuate the building.

There are some general principles to follow:

- If the fire is small and you have a fire blanket or fire extinguisher, you can try to put out the fire, but do not try for longer than 30 seconds.
- If the fire has taken hold, do not try to put it out, do not use lifts, close all doors behind you, and do not open a door without first touching the door handle.
- If a door handle is hot, this indicates that there is a fire behind the door so do not open it but instead find another escape route.
- Walk quickly but do not run.
- If you have to cross a smoke-filled area, stay close to the ground where there will be the least smoke.
- If trapped by a fire, go into a room with a window and shut the door. Open the window and shout for help. If you are able to reach the ground outside the building from the window, escape by going out feet first and lowering yourself onto the ground.
- Call the emergency services as soon as possible.

If a person's clothes are on fire you should STOP, DROP, WRAP and ROLL:

- **STOP** the person from moving around, as this will make the fire worse
- **DROP** the person to the ground
- **WRAP** the person in a non-flammable material
- **ROLL** the person slowly along the ground to extinguish the flames.

key skills

If a person's clothes are on fire, remember STOP, DROP, WRAP and ROLL.

water

Water features in many of our holidays. The main dangers relating to rescue from water result from the fact that the water may be cold, deep and there may be strong underwater currents. Therefore, when attempting to rescue someone from water it is very important that you do not put yourself at risk. It is best to rescue from the water's edge, making sure that you do not get pulled into the water. You can throw a rope or float to a person, or reach out with a stick or branch if you are close to the edge.

If you have to go into the water, wade rather than swim, and do not go out of your depth. Make sure the person's head is out of the water and then drag him to the side. Do not lift the person unnecessarily. Try to shield him from cold wind to prevent any further hypothermia.

electricity

When visiting another country, you should familiarize yourself with the different electricity provision and take with you the necessary adaptors. You must also be aware of the safety of the electrical supply because the majority of injuries caused by an electric current are due to faulty switches or appliances.

If someone is electrocuted, don't touch him until all the electricity is off because if you contact the current you too will be electrocuted. If possible, switch off the electricity. If this is not possible, separate the person from the electrical source. To do this, stand on some dry insulating material such as a book or folded newspaper then, using something made of wood such as a broom, push the electrical source away from the person or the person away from the source. If this is still not possible, carefully loop some rope around the person's ankles and pull him away from the source.

***one-minute** wonder*

Q Can I use a metal pole to isolate the person from the electricity?

A Unfortunately, metal will conduct electricity and you will receive a shock. You must use a material that does not conduct electricity.

***one-minute** wonder*

Q Is it safe to deal with a person under an electricity pylon?

A No. Everyone must stay at least 18 m away from high voltage electricity because it can arc from this distance. The power must be switched off before approaching the person.

key skills

Do not take unacceptable risks when responding to a first-aid situation. You are no use to an injured person if you end up as a victim yourself.

managing an incident

It is important to adopt a systematic approach to any emergency in order to give people the best chance of survival. Be clear in your mind about how to use bystanders, how to access the emergency services, and how to assess the people for injuries. Most first-aid situations, in whatever country you are in, are chaotic and so it is important that someone, possibly you, takes control.

assessing the scene for injured people

Make sure that you know how many people are involved. Check the quiet people first because they may be unconscious and will need your attention first. You can be sure that if a person is shouting or crying out in pain, he is not unconscious. Ask helpers to remove from the scene any people with minor injuries in order to improve access to those who have serious injuries.

Perform primary surveys (see opposite) on any unconscious people first. Treat conscious people with serious injuries, and only then treat conscious people with minor injuries.

the primary survey

The aim of the primary survey is to establish whether the person is conscious and breathing so that you can decide if life-saving first aid is needed. Making sure it is safe to do so, first find out whether the person is conscious or unconscious. You do this by shouting loudly at the person – if you know his name, use it. If you are assessing an adult, you can shake the shoulders gently; if dealing with a child, you should tap the shoulder, and if you are dealing with an infant, you should tap the sole of the foot. If the person is unconscious and you have not already shouted for help, do that now. Then you should open the airway. To do this, place one hand on the forehead and gently tilt the head back. This will make the mouth fall open so that you can look for any obvious obstruction to the airway in or around the mouth and, if present, remove it. Then place two fingers under the point of the chin and lift. This will open the airway. If you are dealing with an infant under one year of age use one finger under the chin.

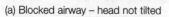

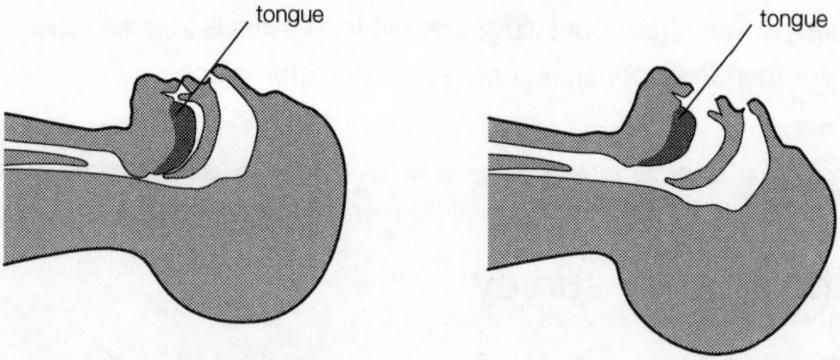

(a) Blocked airway – head not tilted

(b) Unblocked airway – head tilted

Fig 2 Importance of an open airway

With the airway open, you can now check to see if the person is breathing. Do this by putting your head down over his mouth and nose. Look, listen and feel for breathing for around ten seconds. If the person is breathing, you will see the chest moving up and down, you will feel the person's breath on your cheek, and you will hear the sound of the breathing.

If the person is breathing, you should look for any other life-threatening injuries such as severe bleeding. If there is severe bleeding, you will be able to see it without searching around and moving the person. If severe bleeding is present, you should deal with it (see page 30). If there are no other life-threatening injuries, the safest position for the person to be in is the recovery position (see page 41).

Before turning the person into the recovery position, however, you should consider whether or not there is likely to be an injury to the neck. To do this, you look at the mechanism of injury. For example, if the person has been thrown from a moving vehicle and hit his head, it is likely there will be a neck injury. In this instance, it may be better to leave the person in the position in which you found him and to maintain the airway using the jaw-thrust technique (see Chapter 6, page 84). If the airway can be maintained using the jaw-thrust technique that is good. If you can't maintain the airway, or the person shows any sign of vomiting, then you must turn him into the recovery position. If you have a helper, you can ask him to steady the head while you turn the person.

***one-minute** wonder*

Q When I am deciding whether or not to turn the person into the recovery position, which takes priority, a possible neck injury or an open and clear airway?

A An open and clear airway. If the person is not breathing you must start resuscitation (see Chapter 3).

the secondary survey

If you have completed the primary survey and decided that no life-saving action is required, you can carry out a secondary survey. The aim of the secondary survey is to find out more about the person's condition so that the correct first aid can be administered.

You should find out more about the incident by asking the person and any bystanders questions. Ask what happened, when it happened, where it happened and, possibly, why it happened.

Find out more about the mechanism of the injury by looking at how the incident occurred. For example, in a car crash if the impact is from the side, injuries are likely to be on that side of the body. If, on holiday, someone dives into the shallow end of a swimming pool and hits his head, he is likely to have a neck injury.

Find out how the person is feeling. He may be able to tell you about an illness and how the illness makes him feel. The best example of this is a diabetic person who can tell you when his blood sugar is low.

Find out more about the person's injuries by examining him and carrying out a head-to-toe survey (see opposite).

the head-to-toe survey

In order not to miss any vital clues about a person's injuries, it is best to be systematic. Start from the head and work down the body to the toes. While you are doing the survey, think about what the likely problems might be, and work with a high level of suspicion. Often it is not possible to make a definite diagnosis without tests which are only available in hospital, but you can suspect an injury or illness and give the correct first-aid treatment.

what has happened?

First of all, gain more information about the problem. Look for external clues such as objects that could have caused injury, and other clues for example:

- a warning bracelet giving medical history
- a card indicating diabetes, allergy or epilepsy
- an inhaler that may indicate asthma
- an auto injector that indicates a possibility of anaphylaxis
- medicines such as Glyceryl TriNitrate (GTN) that indicate a history of angina
- used needles, syringes, bottles or tins of glue.

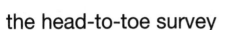

Then look for general signs and symptoms:

- ask the person if he has pain anywhere – if the answer is yes, look at that area for injury
- check the quality of the breathing – it may be fast, slow or laboured — suspect a chest injury
- check the quality of the pulse – it may be fast, slow or irregular – suspect shock
- look at the skin – there may be blueness around the lips – suspect breathing problems
- feel the skin – it may be cold and clammy – suspect shock.

one-minute wonder

Q If I am assessing a person and I find that he has cold clammy skin and a fast, weak pulse what should I suspect?

A Shock. See page 35 for how to treat shock.

Look around the head and neck. If you suspect a neck injury from the mechanism of injury, take care not to move the head. Move your hands carefully over the person's head. Feel for blood which would indicate a scalp wound, or a depression in the skull which would indicate a skull fracture. Look for any blood or yellow fluid coming from the nose or the ears – this is indicative of a fracture of the skull. Look for bleeding, bruising, swelling or a foreign object in the eyes. Look at the pupils. If they are different sizes after a head injury, this indicates cerebral compression – a condition that needs early admission to hospital. Look for swelling, bleeding or bruising around the mouth. Smell the person's breath – alcohol is a common smell. Look at the neck for a medical warning necklace or a stoma (an opening in the neck for breathing – usually after neck surgery). Feel along both collarbones for fractures.

Look at the chest, the back and the abdomen. Ask the person about back pain. If this is accompanied by problems moving the legs, numbness or tingling, do not allow the person to move in case there is a serious back injury that may lead to paralysis. Look at the chest for wounds. Ask the person to take a deep breath, and watch the movement. If there is unequal movement, there may be a chest injury. Listen for wheezing, which may indicate asthma. Look for wounds, swelling, bruising or bleeding around the chest or abdomen. Feel the abdomen for any tenderness or muscle tightness – this may indicate an internal injury. Look for incontinence – the person may have had a seizure. Feel the pelvis for deformity, which may indicate a fracture.

Examine the limbs. Look for any wounds, swelling, bruising, bleeding or deformity. Look for needle marks – this may indicate that the person is an insulin dependent diabetic or possibly an intravenous drug user. Look for a medical warning bracelet. Look at the nails for blueness – this may show that the person is cold.

key skills

Look at the scene of the accident for any clues about the injuries a person may have received. Work slowly and methodically from the head to the toe of the person to detect any abnormalities.

monitoring vital signs

Having carried out the primary and secondary surveys to assess whether or not life-saving measures are required and to try to find out the problem, and having given the correct first-aid treatment, you should take some baseline measurements of breathing, pulse and level of response while waiting for the emergency services to arrive. If possible, you should take these measurements regularly and record them because they can be used to monitor whether the person's condition is getting better or worse.

how to take the pulse

1 There are three places where you can take the pulse. To take the pulse at the wrist, place two fingers at the base of the thumb just below the wrist creases.

2 To take the pulse in the neck, place two fingers on the side of the person's neck between the windpipe and the large muscle in the neck.

3 With babies, take the pulse in the upper arm. Place two fingers on the inner side of the arm at the midpoint between the shoulder and the elbow.

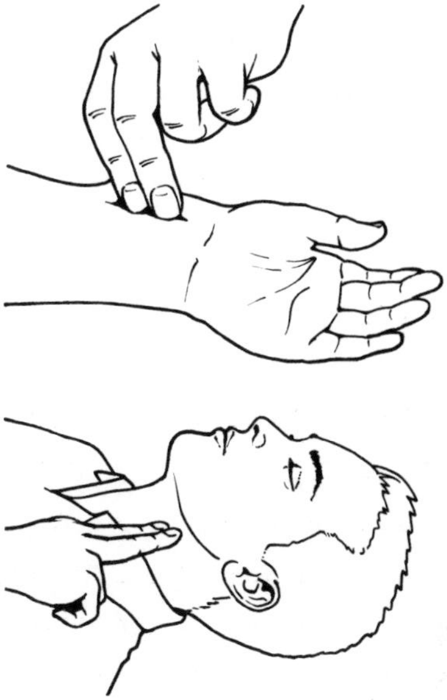

(a) By the wrist

(a) By the neck

Fig 3 Taking the pulse

Assess whether the pulse is:

- fast or slow
- weak or strong
- regular or irregular.

The normal rate in an average adult is between 60 and 80 beats per minute, and in babies it can be up to 140 beats per minute.

one-minute wonder

Q Is it only possible to find a pulse in the wrist and neck of an adult?

A No. There are pulse points at various parts of the body. However, the wrist and the neck are the easiest ones to locate.

how to check the breathing

Listen to the person's breaths and watch the chest rise and fall. Try to do this without the person realizing because we are all able to voluntarily control our breathing. Listen for wheezing or breathing difficulties.

Assess whether the breathing is:

- fast or slow
- deep or shallow
- easy
- difficult or painful.

The normal rate in an average adult is between 12 and 16 breaths per minute, and in babies it can be up to 30 breaths per minute.

how to check the level of response

To check the person's level of response, use the **AVPU** system:

Alert – is the person alert and responding normally to your conversation? If the answer is yes, he is said to be alert and fully conscious.

Verbal – is the person not fully alert but responding to voice and answering simple questions? If the answer is yes, he is said to be responding verbally.

Pain – does the person not respond to voice but respond to pain? If the answer is yes, he is said to respond to pain.

Unconscious – is the person unresponsive to any stimuli? If the answer is yes, he is unconscious.

Other things to watch out for when dealing with an emergency include the dangers of cross-infection, severe blood loss, the presence of shock, and the anxiety you will feel when the emergency is over. We deal with these factors below.

the dangers of cross-infection

In any situation when you are dealing with another person, there is a potential risk of transferring infective organisms such as viruses and bacteria from one person to another. This is especially true when dealing with body fluids, particularly blood and other body fluids contaminated with blood.

It is therefore wise to take some simple precautions:

- wash your hands if possible before and after contact with each person
- wear disposable gloves if possible and if you do not have gloves you can cover your hands with clean plastic bags; but if gloves are not available do not hold back from life saving
- use the person's own hands to put pressure on a bleeding wound
- cover any wounds you have on your hands with waterproof dressings
- try to avoid blood splashes in your eyes or mouth; if you are splashed in the eye, nose, mouth or in a skin wound, wash thoroughly and seek advice from your doctor
- use a plastic bag to dispose of any soiled rubbish and tie it securely at the top.

anxiety when the emergency is over

An emergency is a distressing experience for everyone involved. When you are dealing with the problems, you will be active and focused on what you are doing. However, when it is over and the emergency services have taken people to hospital and cleared up, you are likely to start asking yourself questions.

These may include:

- Did I do the correct things?
- Did I phone for help early enough?
- Did I get enough help from the bystanders?
- What will happen to the injured people?

To ask yourself these questions is normal behaviour, and you must realize that you will feel uncertain and anxious about what happened and what you did to help. Everyone involved is likely to feel this way, including any medical and emergency services staff. You may also feel angry and sad if the outcome of the emergency is poor and if people have died.

It is good to talk and, to help you to face up to your emotions, you should talk about how you feel with a friend or colleague. It would be beneficial to talk to someone who was also involved in the emergency so that you can share feelings. Confidentiality is important, so do not identify people involved in the emergency by name or other personal identification, but there is no reason why you cannot talk about your feelings.

If you release your feelings soon after the emergency, you will probably be able to cope more easily than if you keep your feelings bottled up. Nevertheless, you may still experience feelings of anxiety for some time after the event.

These could include:

- flashbacks of what happened
- nightmares or disturbed sleep
- sweating and tremors
- nausea, especially when thinking about what happened
- tension and irritability
- feelings of isolation and lack of self-confidence.

If you continue to suffer from any of these problems, you should ask for help from your doctor.

key skills

After a first-aid incident, talk to friends and family. Be honest and open, but do not disclose personal details of anyone involved.

summary

If you are the first person on the scene of any emergency situation:

- don't walk by
- get involved
- try and remain calm
- carry out an initial assessment of the airway, breathing and circulation
- talk and listen to the injured person, giving lots of reassurance
- take charge and ask bystanders to help until the emergency services arrive
- dial 999 (or 112 in Europe) for the emergency services
- do not take unacceptable risks.

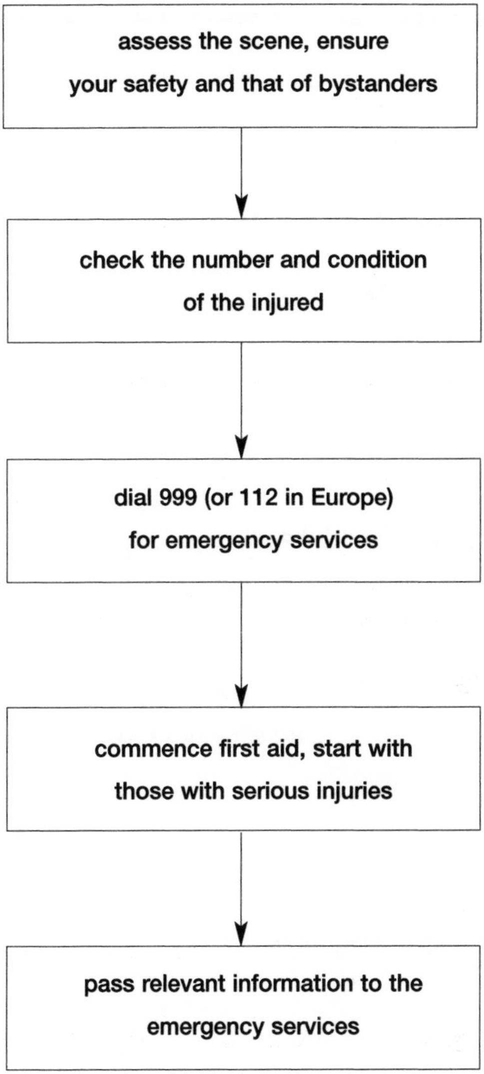

On approaching an emergency situation

self-testers

1 Which emergency services can you access by dialling 999 in the UK?

a fire service
b gas utility service
c NHS Direct
d fell rescue service
e ambulance service

2 Which of the following dangers will stop you from approaching an emergency?

a toxic fumes
b swimming pool full of water
c bomb blast
d stationary vehicles
e falling masonry

3 When you are monitoring a casualty's level of response, what do these letters stand for?

A
V
P
U

4 Which of the following will reduce the chance of cross-infection?

a washing your hands after dealing with a person

b putting a waterproof dressing on a cut on your hand

c avoiding splashes of blood getting in your eye

d wearing disposable gloves

e disposing of all soiled rubbish in a sealed plastic bag

answers

1 **a**, **d** and **e**

2 **a**, **c** and **e**

3 **A**lert, **V**erbal, **P**ain, **U**nconscious

4 **a**, **b**, **c**, **d** and **e**

2

blood loss and shock

If bleeding is severe, it can be dramatic and distressing, especially if there is a large wound somewhere on the body causing the bleeding. The severity of the bleeding depends on the location, size and depth of the wound. Some parts of the body appear to bleed heavily when in fact the actual blood loss is not significant. This applies particularly to the scalp, which has a large network of small blood vessels; when there is even just a small cut to the scalp, there may appear to a lot of blood. If, on the other hand, a person suffers from varicose veins, a very small tear of the vein will lead to copious blood loss, and this may be life threatening if not properly and promptly treated. In this section we focus on blood loss outside the body, but it is also worth remembering that internal bleeding may also occur without any sign of blood – this makes it difficult to diagnose (see page 32).

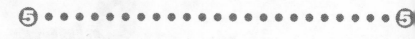

bleeding

When treating a severe bleed, your aims are to:

- stop the bleeding as quickly as possible
- prevent the onset of shock
- minimize the risk of infection.

To stop the bleeding, quickly place pressure directly on the wound using your hand, the person's hand or a clean pad, if available. At the same time, raise the injured limb above the level of the heart. This helps to reduce the blood flow to the wound by using gravity and ensuring that all the essential organs are kept adequately supplied with blood.

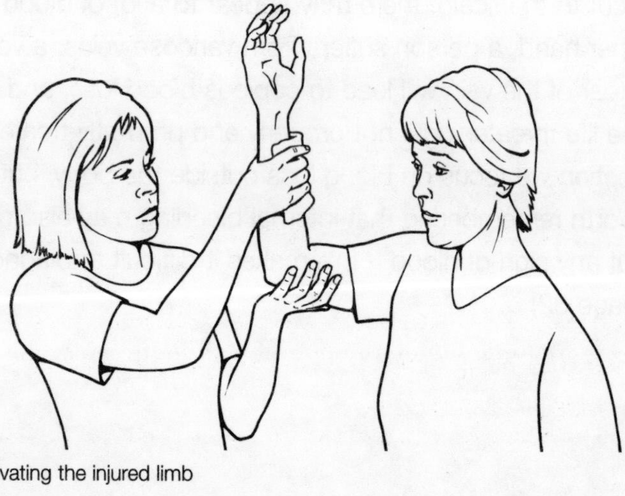

Fig 4 Elevating the injured limb

In the event of a leg wound, it is important to help the person to lie down and elevate the leg above the level of the heart. If the injury is on the arm, the person should sit down and elevate the arm. Once it is elevated, secure a pad or dressing in place, ensuring that pressure is maintained.

You may have been taught that if you are caring for a severe bleed you should apply a tourniquet in the form of a tie or a narrow piece of clothing around the affected limb. This is no longer a recommended first-aid procedure because it has been proven that to stem the blood supply to the wound you do not necessarily have to cut off the blood supply to the whole of the limb.

key skills

To treat a serious bleed, apply pressure to the wound. If the wound is on a limb, elevate the limb above the level of the heart. Call for an ambulance and continue to reassure the person.

one-minute wonder

Q Should I apply direct pressure on the wound first or should I elevate it?

A Both pressure and elevation are effective ways to stop the bleeding. It is not important which of these you do first, provided that you do both.

Many severe bleeds are caused by glass or knives or other sharp objects that may be embedded in the wound. It is crucial to have a quick look to see if there is anything embedded in the wound. If there is, you should not remove it because the object may be helping to stem the blood flow; by removing it you may cause further internal damage and make it bleed more. To treat a wound with an embedded object, apply pressure to the edges of the wound and bandage around the object. Make sure that you do not apply direct pressure to the object. Ensure that the person has immediate medical attention because the object will need to be removed in a surgical procedure and the resulting wound treated accordingly.

Severe bleeding can result in shock (see page 34). You must monitor the person for signs of shock, and treat them accordingly.

internal bleeding

As mentioned above, it can be very difficult to diagnose internal bleeding. However, the things you should consider if you suspect this type of bleeding are: the history of the incident, what has happened – has something fallen on to the person? Has the person fallen onto something? Has there been an impact (in particular to the abdomen)? The abdominal area is particularly vulnerable in the case of an impact and as it houses many of the body's key organs, it is particularly susceptible to internal bleeding with life-threatening implications if not diagnosed. If you suspect internal bleeding, look at the area. Take into account the history of what has happened. Does the person appear to be going into shock? If so, is this disproportionate to the injuries you can see? Is the person breathing more rapidly? Is the person's pulse rate increasing? Is there evidence of bruising and is the area tender? You also need to remember that blood may be visible. However, as mentioned, the blood loss you see externally may be disproportionate to the shock the injured person is experiencing.

If you suspect internal bleeding, help the person to lie down, raise the legs, loosen any tight clothing, especially around the abdomen, get help as early as possible and continue to monitor the person until such time as the ambulance arrives.

nose bleed

To treat a nose bleed you should sit the person down leaning forward, pinch the soft part of the nose and keep the nose pinched for ten minutes. If, after ten minutes, the bleeding has not stopped, pinch the nose for two further periods of ten minutes. Once bleeding has stopped, clean around the nose and mouth and allow the person to rest. If the nose bleed lasts longer than 30 minutes arrange for the person to be taken to hospital.

shock

Shock is a term used to describe a range of situations from feelings of anxiety to a serious clinical state in which the body has lost a lot of blood or body fluids. It is important to be aware of the differences. In all emergency situations, there will be a feeling of shock and anxiety about what has happened. This feeling will be severe amongst all involved if it has been a serious incident with many injured people. Here we deal with clinical shock rather than with the shock that is an emotional response to something you've seen or heard.

Clinical shock is the body's physical response to a condition or injury. It is a life-threatening state in which the circulating fluid in the body is reduced and organs such as the heart and brain do not get enough blood. As a consequence, there is not enough oxygen and nutrients for them to function properly. Clinical shock is most commonly the result of blood loss, but it can be caused by fluid loss, for example, in burns.

If you suspect shock, you should look for:

- an injury or illness leading to the shock
- pale, cold, clammy skin
- restlessness
- yawning and sighing
- nausea

- thirst
- rapid and then weak pulse
- fast and shallow breathing
- gradual loss of consciousness.

To help a person in shock, you should treat the underlying problem, if possible. Help the person to lie down. Reassure him constantly as he will be very anxious. Raise the person's legs above the level of the heart so that the blood in the legs flows down towards the heart and the brain where it is most needed. Keep the person warm by covering him with a light blanket, but be careful because overheating will make the shock worse. Monitor and record the vital signs – pulse, breathing and level of response – regularly until help arrives. Do not give the person anything to eat or drink because further treatment requiring an anaesthetic may be necessary in hospital.

one-minute wonder

Q Is it true that a hot drink (such as sweet tea) helps someone in shock?

A It may be helpful to a person with anxiety, but not if the person has clinical shock. It is preferable not to give him anything to eat or drink.

key skills

Clinical shock is a very dangerous condition. You must help the injuried person to lie down, treat the cause, raise the legs, and keep the person warm.

summary

The loss of a large amount of blood from the body can be life threatening. Your aim as a first aider is to reduce or stop the amount of blood leaving the body while ensuring the wound, if it is external bleeding, is kept as clean as possible.

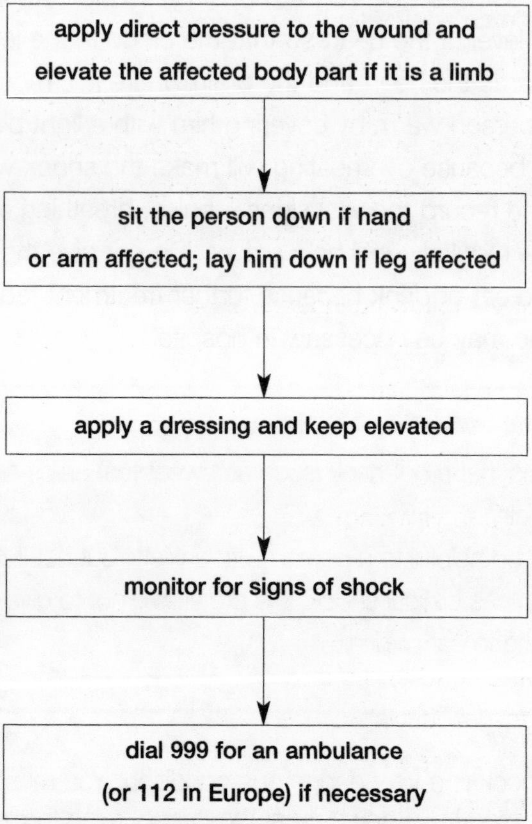
apply direct pressure to the wound and elevate the affected body part if it is a limb
sit the person down if hand or arm affected; lay him down if leg affected
apply a dressing and keep elevated
monitor for signs of shock
dial 999 for an ambulance (or 112 in Europe) if necessary

How to treat severe external bleeding

self-testers

1 To treat a nose bleed you should:

a sit the person forward and pinch the nose

b tilt the head back and pinch the nose

c lay the person down and elevate their legs

d tilt the head forward and let the blood drain out

2 To treat internal bleeding you should:

a lay the person down and elevate their legs

b sit the person upright and loosen any tight clothing

c lay the person down, raise their legs and loosen any tight clothing, especially around the abdomen

d place the person in the recovery position

3 Which of the following indicate shock?

a cold, clammy skin

b strong, slow pulse

c thirst

d slow breathing

e sighing and yawning

4 To treat shock you should:

a take the person's clothes off

b raise the head and shoulders

c treat the underlying cause

d stand the person up

e raise the legs

answers

1 **a**

2 **a** and **c**

3 **a**, **c** and **e**

4 **c** and **e**

3

how to resuscitate

Finding a person who is collapsed and needs resuscitation is a frightening experience, but it is important to try to remain calm and to think clearly. This may happen anywhere from the top of a mountain to a crowded piazza. It is also likely to happen to a travelling companion or a relative. (If you are travelling abroad it is always good to know how to call for the emergency services in that country.) You should know when to call an ambulance, and be ready to give the ambulance service personnel an indication of the emergency of the situation. If the person is not breathing, you will need to breathe for him. If there are no signs of heart activity, you will need to do chest compressions.

In this chapter, you will learn when to call for an ambulance, how to check for response, how to check for breathing, and how to do chest compressions. In Chapter 1, you were given information about the dangers that you might encounter in an emergency situation, and so in this chapter it is assumed that any danger has been dealt with.

how to check for a response

To check for a response, talk to the person and gently shake his shoulders. If dealing with a child, do not shake in case you cause an injury. If dealing with a baby, tap the sole of the foot. If there is no response, shout for help and check if the airway is open. If it is not, open the airway as described in Chapter 1, page 11.

one-minute wonder

Q People often talk of swallowing the tongue. What does this mean?

A The tongue is not actually swallowed but, when you lose consciousness, you also lose muscle tone and, if you are lying on your back, the tongue can flop into the back of the throat and block the airway. When you tip the head back, the tongue regains its normal position on the floor of the mouth.

If the person is breathing, look for any other life-threatening problems such as visible severe bleeding, and deal with those. Then place the person in the recovery position (see opposite).

the recovery position

The recovery position is the safest position for an unconscious person. It ensures that the tongue does not block the airway, that any vomit drains from the mouth and, if there is any blood, that this does not stop the person breathing. The chest can move freely making breathing as easy as possible. The position is stable.

To put a person into the recovery position, kneel beside him. Remove spectacles and any bulky objects from the pocket on the side you are going to roll the person on to. Place the arm that is nearest to you at a right angle to the person's body. Bend the elbow and face the palm upwards. Bring the other arm across his body and hold the back of this hand to his cheek. With your other hand, grasp the person's far leg just above the knee and pull it up until the foot is flat on the floor. Pull on the far leg and roll him towards you. Adjust the upper leg so that it is at right angles at the hip and the knee. Tilt the head back to make sure the airway stays open. For a baby aged less than one year, hold him in your arms with his head lower than his body and his face towards you.

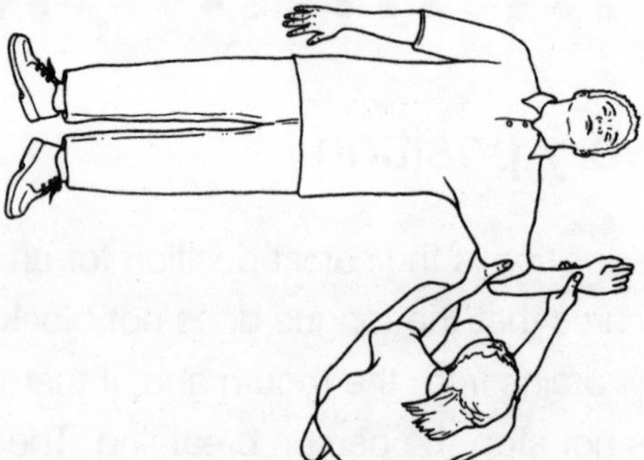

(a) Place the arm nearest to you at a right angle to the person's body.

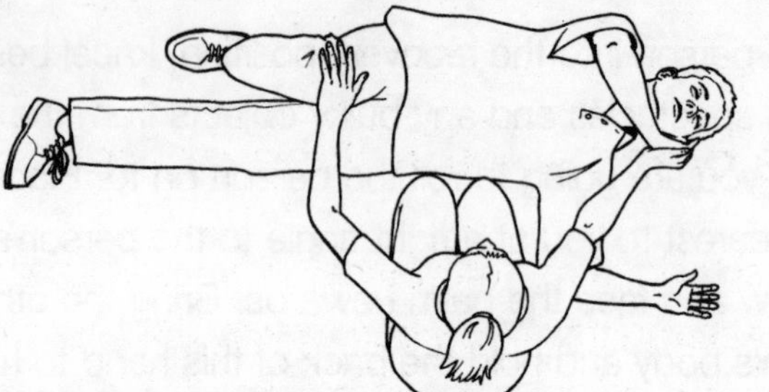

(b) Place the other hand, palm outwards, against the person's cheek. Pull up the far knee until the foot is flat on the floor.

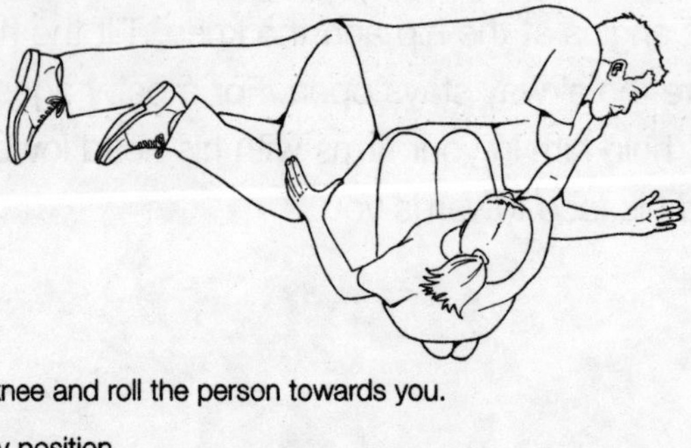

(c) Pull on the far knee and roll the person towards you.

Fig 5 The recovery position

one-minute wonder

Q If I have to go to a telephone to get help, is it safe to leave the person?

A Make the person as safe as you possibly can by putting him into the recovery position.

If the person is not breathing, call for emergency help and give two rescue breaths (see below).

5 • 5

rescue breaths – the 'kiss of life'

To give rescue breaths, follow these instructions and see Figure 6. Keeping the airway open, pinch the nose and place your mouth around the person's mouth. Blow steadily until the chest rises – you will see this out of the corner of your eye. Then take your mouth away and watch the chest fall. If the chest rises as you blow, and falls as you take your mouth away, you have given an effective breath. For an adult, the rate of rescue breathing is every six seconds. For a child or baby, the rate of rescue breathing is every three seconds.

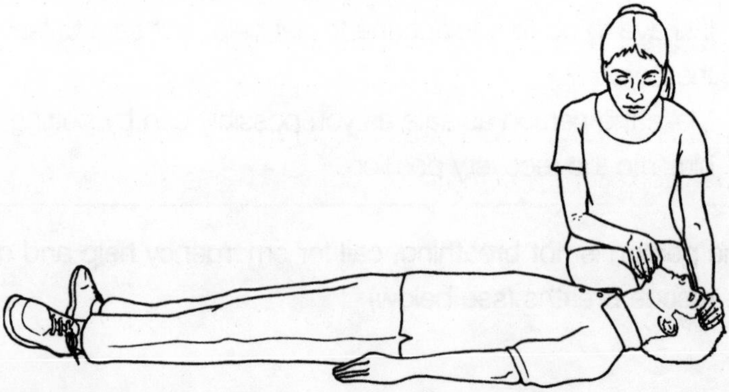

(a) Place one hand on the forehead and your fingertips under the chin and gently tilt the head back.

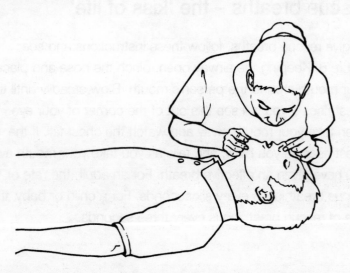

(b) Pinch the nose, place your mouth over the person's mouth and blow.

Fig 6 How to give rescue breaths

Having called for emergency help and given two effective rescue breaths, check whether the person shows any signs of blood circulation. The signs are breathing, coughing or movement of the body or limbs. Take a quick look for no longer than ten seconds. If there are no signs, you should try to provide some artificial blood circulation by doing chest compressions (see below).

key skills

The assessment of an injured person should be based on DR ABC:

- **D**anger
- **R**esponse
- **A**irway
- **B**reathing
- **C**irculation.

5 5

chest compressions – 'chest pumps'

To perform chest compressions, kneel beside the person and find the lower half of the breastbone. Do this by using your middle finger of one hand to find the point where the lowermost rib meets the breastbone. Place your index finger on the breastbone beside your middle finger, run the heel of your other hand down the breastbone and place it next to the fingers.

This is the point you apply pressure. Place the heel of one of your hands on the breastbone. Then place the heel of your other hand on top and interlock your fingers. Lean over the person and, keeping your arms straight, press down by about 4–5 cm or 1.5–2 inches at a rate of 100 per minute. For a child, use one hand and press down one third of the depth of the chest. For a baby, use two fingers and press down one third of the depth of the chest. Release the pressure without taking your hands off the chest.

If the person is still unconscious with no signs of breathing or cirulation, perform cardio pulmonary resuscitation (CPR) by combining chest compressions with rescue breaths at a ratio of two breaths to 15 chest compressions (see Figure 7). Continue CPR until help arrives and takes over, you are so exhausted you cannot carry on, or the person takes a breath or makes a movement. In a remote setting it is difficult to know whether to go for help or start resuscitation. You can attract attention by shouting, blowing a whistle or sending up a flare, but if there is no prospect of being able to call for help, it is probably best to start CPR. Carry on for as long as you can as someone else might come along to help you. This action gives the person the best chance of survival, and you will feel as though you have done something to help.

key skills

If a person is unconscious with no signs of breathing or circulation, you should deliver two rescue breaths followed by 15 compressions. Continue this cycle until help arrives.

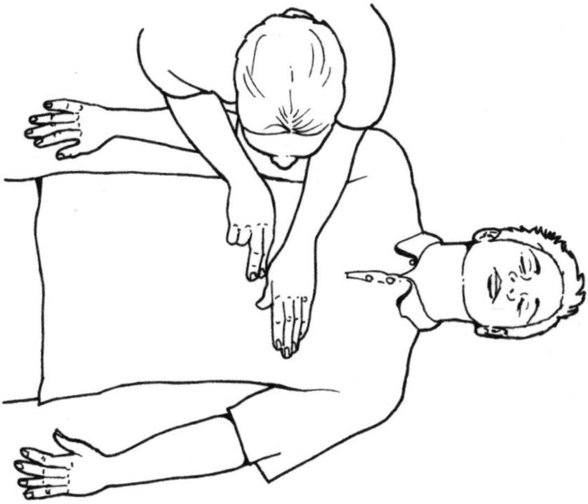

(a) Place your middle finger and index finger on the lower half of the breastbone.

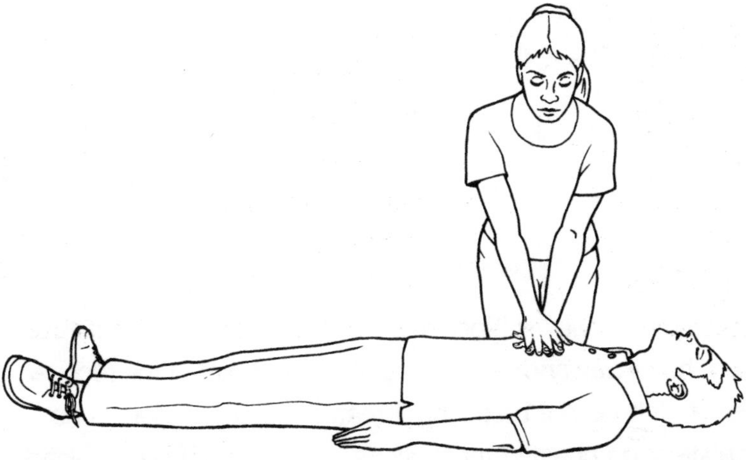

(b) Run the heel of your hand down the breastbone to your fingers. Place the heel of your other hand on top and interlock your fingers. Keep your arms straight and use the heel to press down.

Fig 7 How to perform chest compressions

one-minute wonder

Q Will I damage the heart if there is still a faint heartbeat and I do chest compressions?

A This is a very small risk, but the benefits of doing chest compressions in this situation very much outweigh that risk.

one-minute wonder

Q Will I restart the heart by doing chest compressions?

A This is unlikely – to restart the heart you need a defibrillator, a machine that sends an electrical charge across the heart to try to restart it. By doing chest compressions, you are maintaining some blood circulation while waiting for the emergency services to bring a defibrillator. It is also worth remembering that defibrillators are accessible to the public, especially in airports, train stations and shopping centres. They should only be operated by trained staff.

summary

If a person's airway is blocked, it makes breathing very difficult. Open the airway and, if he is breathing, put him in the recovery position. If he is not breathing, breathe for him. If there is no circulation, do chest compressions. If there is still no circulation and no signs of breathing, do CPR.

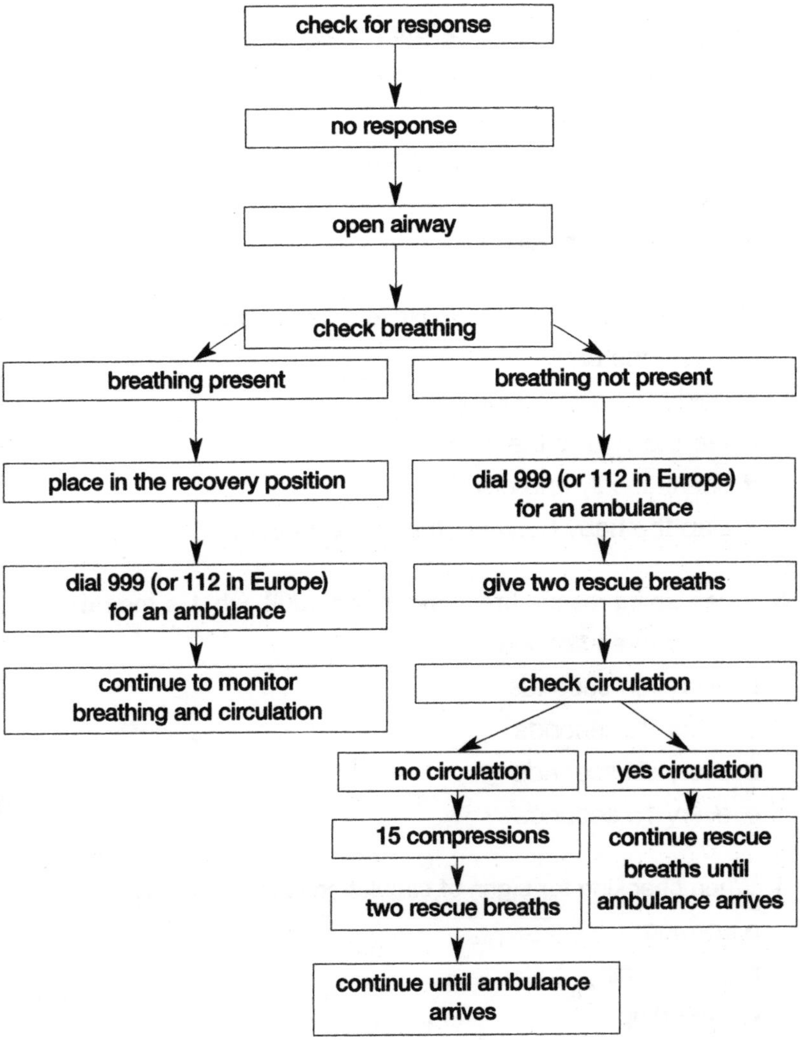

How to assess an unconscious person

self-testers

1 The recovery position is a safe position because:

a if the person is sick, the vomit will drain away
b the airway stays open
c the tongue doesn't drop back into the throat
d the chest can move freely
e it is a stable position

2 When checking for a response in a baby, what should you do?

a shake the baby
b hold the baby upside down
c tap the sole of the baby's foot
d speak loudly and clearly
e slap the baby between the shoulder blades

3 When doing rescue breathing for an adult, what is the rate?

a every three seconds
b every ten seconds
c every 20 seconds
d every six seconds
e every 15 seconds

4 When checking for signs of circulation what should you look for?

a moving
b eye opening
c breathing
d coughing
e colour of the skin

5 What is the ratio for rescue breaths to chest compressions for an adult?

a 2:15
b 1:5
c 3:12
d 5:50
e 2:10

6 What is the rate for chest compressions?

a varies for babies and children
b is 100 per minute for all ages
c depends on the size of the person
d 80 per minute for all ages
e depends on how fast you can do them

---

answers

1 **a**, **b**, **c**, **d** and **e**
2 **c** and **d**
3 **d**
4 **a**, **b**, **c** and **d**
5 **a**
6 **b**

4

hot climates

Exposure to the sun: travelling in hot climates can lead to some specific conditions. There are a number of actions that you can take to help prevent these conditions such as avoiding too much contact with direct sunlight, regularly cooling down in the shade or sea, ensuring that you keep yourself hydrated, and avoiding over-demanding activities at the hottest time of the day.

sunburn

Sunburn is a constant outdoor hazard in a hot climate and can contribute to dehydration and heat exhaustion. Wearing light clothing and frequently applying high factor sunscreen can prevent it. At high altitude, sunburn can happen without exposure to direct sunlight.

how to recognize sunburn

The signs of sunburn are:

- red skin
- pain in the area of the red skin
- blistering of the skin.

action to take

If you suspect sunburn, take the person out of the sun and into a cool shady place. Cool the skin by splashing or sponging with cool water. Give the person frequent sips of water to drink to prevent dehydration (see Chapter 6, page 74). If the sunburn is mild, it can be soothed by calamine lotion or after-sun cream. If the skin is severely blistered, seek medical help if possible.

one-minute wonder

Q Is sunburn the same as sunstroke?

A No. Sunstroke is covered in this chapter under the more commonly known name of heat stroke. Guidance on the treatment for sunstroke can be found on page 57.

prickly heat

Prickly heat is a sweat rash that is common on arrival in a hot, humid climate. It occurs particularly on parts of the body from which sweat cannot evaporate, such as the feet. It can be avoided by dressing correctly until acclimatized to the heat.

how to recognize prickly heat

The signs of prickly heat are:

- tiny red spots or blisters
- prickly or burning sensation on the site of the rash.

action to take

To treat prickly heat, cool the skin by either sponging it or showering it with cool water. Apply calamine lotion if you have it.

polymorphic light eruption

This is an immune reaction to the sun's UVA rays and follows exposure to very strong sunlight. It is especially common in women and is often confused with prickly heat. Some people suffer from it every time they are exposed to strong sunlight and are therefore advised to take precautions such as phasing in exposure to the sun.

how to recognize polymorphic light eruption (PLE)

You can recognize if the person has polymorphic light eruption PLE by an itchy, spotty rash, often over the upper body.

action to take

Use sunscreens with high anti-UVA protection and avoid other creams and cosmetics.

heat exhaustion

This is caused by an abnormally high loss of water and salt from the body through excessive sweating.

how to recognize heat exhaustion

The signs of heat exhaustion are:

- headache and confusion
- sweating and pale, clammy skin
- muscle cramps
- rapid, weak pulse
- weak breathing.

action to take

If a person is suffering from heat exhaustion, help him into a shady place and ask him to lie down and raise his legs if possible. Give water or rehydration sachets in small amounts frequently until he recovers. If he loses consciousness, put him into the recovery position (see page 41) and seek help.

heat stroke

Heat stroke (or sunstroke) is caused by a failure of the normal temperature regulating mechanism in the brain. It can follow dehydration and heat exhaustion – when sweating stops, the body cannot be cooled by sweat evaporation. The body becomes dangerously overheated and the person can lose consciousness quickly, so it is important to act immediately to get the temperature down.

how to recognize heat stroke

The signs of heat stroke are:

- the body feels very hot, flushed and dry
- the temperature is above 40°C
- headache, dizziness and confusion
- full, rapid pulse
- rapid loss of consciousness.

action to take

If you suspect heat stroke, you must act quickly to move the person to a cool place. Remove the person's outer clothing and, if possible, pour cool water over him or fan him with clothing. Alternatively, wrap the person in a cold, wet sheet or clothing, and get emergency help. If he loses consciousness, place him in the recovery position (see page 41) and be ready to resuscitate.

one-minute wonder

Q Rehydration salt sachets are heavy to carry when I am out walking? Do I really need them?

A In the initial stages of hot climate problems frequent sips of water are probably more important than salts. Salt replacement comes later.

key skills

For travel in hot climates:

- use sunscreen
- wear light clothing
- phase in exposure to strong sunlight
- watch out for heatstroke and prevent if possible.

summary

For most heat-related conditions, you should keep the person cool, take him out of sunlight and cool his skin with water. Give sips of water to drink. These conditions can become serious if not treated quickly.

self-testers

1 Actions to take to try to relieve sunburn include:

a giving a long, cold drink
b cooling the skin with cool water
c giving frequent sips of water
d applying after-sun cream
e staying in the sun

2 The signs of heat exhaustion include:

a headache
b pale, clammy skin
c slow pulse
d deep breathing
e sweating

3 Actions to relieve heat exhaustion include:

a asking the person to run around to cool down
b giving a long, cold drink
c avoiding rehydration products
d staying in the sun
e lying the person down and raising his legs

4 Features of PLE include:

a it is common in women
b it occurs mainly on the legs
c it is caused by very strong sun
d it is prevented by the use of anti-UVA creams
e it is made worse by some cosmetics

5 The signs of heat stroke include:

a a slow, shallow pulse
b pale, clammy skin
c headache and confusion
d hot, flushed skin
e sweating

6 Heat stroke is relieved by:

a keeping the clothes on
b wrapping in a cool, wet sheet
c removing outer clothing
d maintaining activity
e staying in the sun

---

answers

1 **b**, **c** and **d**
2 **a**, **b** and **e**
3 **e**
4 **a**, **c**, **d** and **e**
5 **c** and **d**
6 **b** and **c**

5

cold climates

It is easy to overlook the effects of travel in a cold climate and to be unprepared for the extremes of cold and wind that can occur. It is especially important to take into account wind chill factors.

When travelling in a cold climate, you can take some measures to prevent suffering the effects of extreme cold. For example:

- research the climate where you are going
- tell someone where you are going
- wear good insulating waterproof clothing
- wear a hat and gloves
- wear good waterproof boots
- take some equipment with you such as a foil blanket, spare clothing or blankets
- take warm drinks and high-energy food such as chocolate
- if the conditions are snowy, wear sunglasses or goggles. Always be prepared for the worst possible conditions.

hypothermia

Hypothermia is a condition in which the body temperature falls below 35°C. The effects vary according to how far and how quickly the temperature falls. Hypothermia is caused by exposure to cold. When out of doors, the 'wind chill' factor plays a big part in the speed at which hypothermia develops because the body cools faster in moving air than in still air. Hypothermia is also caused by immersion in cold water. In this circumstance, the effects of hypothermia appear very quickly because the body cools 30 times faster in water. Fatigue, alcohol, drugs and chronic illness can all contribute to the development of hypothermia.

one-minute wonder

Q You mention that alcohol can contribute to the development of hypothermia. How?

A Alcohol can be a contributing factor because it affects the circulation by dilating the blood vessels in the skin and increasing heat loss from the body. There are no medical benefits of giving a person with hypothermia a shot of whisky.

how to recognize hypothermia

The signs of hypothermia are:

- shivering
- cold, pale, dry skin
- apathy
- disorientation or irrational behaviour
- lethargy
- slow, shallow breathing
- slow, weak pulse leading later to loss of consciousness and possibly cardiac arrest.

action to take

If you suspect hypothermia, your aim as a first aider is to help the person to a sheltered place away from the wind. If his clothing is wet and you have spare clothing or blankets, remove his wet clothing and cover him with the dry clothing and blankets. If you have a dry sleeping bag, use that. Cover his head. Try to insulate the person from the ground using any dry vegetation available. Administer warm drinks if possible as they will raise the temperature of the body but ensure that these drinks are not too hot. Give high-energy food such as chocolate. If you are part of a party, send two people for help. If the person loses consciousness, put him into the recovery position (see page 41). If the person stops breathing and his heart stops, start resuscitation (see Chapter 3).

things you should not do

Do not take off your clothes to give to the other person as this will lead to you losing heat and risking hypothermia. You must not jump into a sleeping bag with a person who is very cold, as this will lead to you losing heat and risking hypothermia. You can help to insulate the person by lying on top of the bag, but take care not to lie too still as you will go to sleep in the cold. Do not go for help if you are alone because the person may lose consciousness at any time. Instead, try to attract attention by blowing a whistle, flashing a torch or lighting a fire. Do not administer alcohol because this dilates the blood vessels in the skin and allows heat to escape from the body, making the hypothermia worse. You must also not stop your resuscitation efforts unless you are absolutely exhausted because later rewarming can restart the heart.

one-minute wonder

Q If there are no spare, dry clothes, should I give the person some of mine?

A It is best not to because you will have to seek help and, if you take off your clothes, you too are at risk of hypothermia.

key skills

warm the person with dry clothing, insulate him from the ground, and give warm drinks or high-energy food. Don't end up with hypothermia yourself.

frostbite

Frostbite is a condition in which the fingers or toes freeze as a result of being exposed to very low temperatures in freezing or cold and windy conditions. In many cases, frostbite is accompanied by hypothermia. Initially the digits feel very cold, but when exposure continues they develop gangrene as the blood vessels become permanently damaged.

how to recognize frostbite

The signs of frostbite are:

- pins and needles in the fingers or toes
- pale skin at first, then later mottled and blue
- numbness
- hardening of the skin
- if gangrene starts, the skin will be blue-black
- on recovery, the skin will be painful, red, hot and possibly blistered.

action to take

If you suspect a person is suffering from frostbite, remove his gloves, boots and other constrictions such as rings. Warm the person's digits with your hands or, if the fingers are involved, put them in the person's armpits. Rewarming will be painful. If the toes are affected, put them in your armpits. Then, place the warmed digits in warm water for at least ten minutes and dry carefully. If you have one, lightly apply a bandage. Elevate the limb to reduce swelling, and give the person a painkiller if the pain is severe. Take the person to hospital for further treatment.

things you should not do

You should not rub the skin because you will damage it. Do not put the digits near direct heat or use hot water because you will rewarm them too fast. Do not allow the person to smoke as this will constrict the blood vessels and make the situation worse. Do not attempt to thaw the digits if there is a likelihood of refreezing.

key skills

Warm the affected digits. Use your heat or the other person's to do this. Give the person a painkiller if available.

trench foot

Trench foot is a type of frostbite caused by prolonged exposure to very low temperatures in damp conditions. Tight shoes, wet socks and lack of mobility aggravate the condition.

how to recognize trench foot

The feet are white, cold, numb and, on rewarming, are red, hot and painful.

action to take

The treatment is the same as for frostbite.

summary

Cold can kill if you do not take action. Warm the person and do not give him alcohol or cigarettes. If the person's breathing and heart stop, be prepared to resuscitate.

self-testers

1 The signs of hypothermia include:

a red skin
b rapid pulse
c slow, weak pulse
d cold, dry skin
e irrational behaviour

2 Help can be given to a hypothermic person by:

a covering over wet clothing
b covering the head
c giving a 'hot toddy'
d giving some chocolate
e insulating from the wet ground

3 What are the things you should not do for hypothermia?

a take off your clothes
b leave the person alone
c give a warm drink
d put the person in a dry sleeping bag
e give an alcoholic drink

4 What is frostbite?

a a condition that mainly affects the hands and feet
b a result of exposure to freezing conditions
c a condition that makes the skin turn mottled and blue
d a condition that is very painful when rewarming takes place
e a condition that is always reversible

5 To treat frostbite, what can you do?

a put the person's feet into your armpits
b put the person's hands into very hot water
c leave the person's fingers wet
d apply a light bandage
e raise the person's limb

6 What should you not do when treating frostbite?

a rub the skin
b put the hands in a bowl of warm water
c give a painkiller if the pain is severe
d allow the person to smoke
e thaw out the fingers when they can possibly refreeze

answers

1 **c**, **d** and **e**

2 **b**, **d** and **e**

3 **a**, **b** and **e**

4 **a**, **b**, **c** and **d**

5 **a**, **d** and **e**

6 **a**, **d** and **e**

6

backpacking

When setting out on a backpacking expedition, most people are concerned about serious problems that might happen such as transport difficulties, tropical diseases and exotic infections. However, the reality is that you are much more likely to be affected by minor injuries and ailments such as blisters, sunburn and insect stings.

Accidents are the leading cause of serious injury abroad. They happen regularly on the road, on and in water, and from falls from hotel balconies. Everyone should be aware of what to do in a serious emergency such as a hostel fire or a car crash (see Chapter 1). The physical demands of backpacking mean that there are some considerations you should make prior to and while you are undertaking your holiday.

Plan your journey in short distances so that the physical demands do not become too great. Use good equipment and don't carry unnecessary items. The backpacking community is a very close one. Speak to fellow travellers about any advice they can share with you to reduce the risk of injury or illness.

before setting out

There are some things that can be done to try to eliminate problems while backpacking. These include equipping yourself with a small, basic first-aid kit. If travelling to a remote area, ask a specialist travel clinic to recommend what you should take in an extended first-aid kit. Before you go, make sure you have the correct immunizations for the part of the world you are visiting and passing through.

Find out if you will be backpacking at altitude, and arrange for time to acclimatize. If you have a common recurring health problem, ensure that you are carrying everything that you need to treat it. You could also attend a personal safety course. Check you have insurance to cover health problems and accidents, and keep notes of phone numbers of people you might need to reach, as well as medical records and important medicines.

one-minute wonder

Q If I am told the water is safe to drink, should I just go ahead and drink it?

A It is probably better to assume the water is not drinkable, especially in a remote area. It is best to choose bottled water and have the bottle opened in your presence. Use bottled water for cleaning teeth and, if you have to use water from the tap, use hot water and allow it to cool. Take water purification tablets with you.

5 • 5

dehydration

Dehydration is common when backpacking, particularly in hot and humid climates. It is made worse by exertion, high altitude, and exposure to the sun for long periods of time. Dehydration is also more likely to occur if you have diarrhoea. Dehydration must be attended to at an early stage to prevent it from leading to heat exhaustion and heat stroke (see Chapter 5, pages 56 and 57).

how to recognize dehydration

The signs of dehydration are:

- thirst
- nausea
- headache
- dizziness
- fatigue
- dark coloured urine
- muscle cramps.

action to take

If a person is dehydrated, go into a shady place if possible and advise the person to drink small, frequent amounts of water until he feels better. If you have oral rehydration sachets containing a solution of sugar and salt you can use them but you must make a very dilute solution and follow the instructions on the sachet. Advise the person to rest until fully recovered.

one-minute wonder

Q Is it true that you can take tablet salt as a cure for dehydration?

A Yes, salt can be taken, but only in a diluted form. You can make your own rehydration solution by adding one teaspoon of salt and four to five teaspoons of sugar to 1 litre of clean drinking water.

diarrhoea

Diarrhoea is a very common problem associated with backpacking. In some parts of the world 80 per cent of travellers may be affected. It is sensible to find out about food hygiene before setting out. Diarrhoea is a result of irritation of the bowel by contaminated food and water, alcohol, unusual or rich foods, or some medicines.

action to take

To treat diarrhoea, give the person frequent sips of water, gradually increasing the amount over time. The person should avoid eating until the appetite comes back, and then eat only bland foods in small quantities. Give anti-diarrhoeal medicines if necessary. If the diarrhoea persists, suspect something more serious such as salmonella infection and seek medical help.

key skills

Be prepared for dehydration and diarrhoea. Drink plenty and take care with food hygiene.

altitude sickness

Altitude sickness is potentially lethal because it can lead to 'waterlogging of the brain and lungs', but it is also preventable. It is easy to overlook altitude when backpacking, so it is important to always check how high you are going.

> ***one-minute wonder***
>
> **Q** How do I prevent altitude sickness?
>
> **A** Allow plenty of time to become accustomed to high altitude and, if ascending overland, do it gradually.

how to recognize altitude sickness

Altitude sickness presents in different individuals in different ways. If it is mild, the signs are:

- breathlessness
- nausea
- headache
- dizziness.

If it is severe, the signs are:

- confusion
- loss of co-ordination
- sleep problems
- wheezing and breathlessness.

action to take

Rest, and advise descent to the last altitude at which the person felt well. If available, help the person to take oxygen. Many travel companies who regularly lead tours at high altitude will carry oxygen with them.

blisters

The persistent rubbing of the skin by something irregular such as ill-fitting boots or rough socks can cause blisters.

how to recognize blisters

A blister may start as a small red spot but, if the friction continues, it becomes a fluid-filled sac under the skin surface and is very painful.

action to take

If the person is not actively walking, do not burst the blister. Instead, pad around it, secure the pad, and the fluid in the sac will gradually be absorbed into the body. If the person is actively walking, clean the area of the blister with clean water and pop the blister. This is advisable as continued walking will pop the blister eventually and, if it is done as a planned procedure, it is possible to keep the area clean and therefore reduce the chance of infection. Apply a protective covering such as a blister plaster, and make sure the covering is fixed securely in place. Also check that the plaster extends beyond the area of the blister.

one-minute wonder

Q Why is a blister plaster better than an ordinary plaster?

A A blister plaster has a cushion of jelly-like material that acts as a 'second skin' when applied. This means there is less chance of it becoming dislodged and causing more rubbing when walking than there is with an ordinary plaster.

cuts and grazes

Minor injuries, cuts and scrapes happen all the time when backpacking and, if they are not kept clean, they will take longer to heal than usual.

how to look after a small wound

Rinse the wound with cool, clean water if possible or use an alcohol-free wipe. Dry thoroughly and apply a dressing that extends beyond the edges of the wound. Leave the dressing in place to allow the wound to heal. If the dressing gets dirty, replace with a clean dressing.

ruises

bruise occurs when an injury breaks blood vessels under the kin. Bruises vary greatly in size and in the length of time they ke to go away.

ow to recognize bruises

he signs of a bruise are:

- painful swelling under the skin
- blue-black colour of the swelling.

ction to take

the bruise is on a limb, raise the limb up to reduce the blood ow to it, and apply firm pressure with a bandage or cloth. If ou can, soak a cloth in cold water and apply this as a cold ompress for at least five minutes. Reapply the compress until e bruise stops getting bigger.

ow to make a cold compress

oak a cloth in cold water. Wring it out, fold it, and place it firmly on the injury. Re-soak the cloth every five minutes to keep it cool. If ere is access to ice cubes, fill a plastic bag with them, wrap in a loth and apply firmly to the injury. Alternatively, you may have a bag f frozen peas or an ice pack. Always wrap a cold pack in a cloth ecause, if applied directly to the skin, it may cause a cold burn.

cramp

Cramp in the muscles of the legs is common, especially after strenuous exercise. It happens when a muscle is stressed repeatedly, and it is caused by a lack of oxygen to the muscle and i made worse by an excessive loss of salt and water from the body through sweating.

how to recognize cramp

The signs of cramp are:

- sudden pain in a muscle
- the muscle feels very tight.

action to take

Breathe deeply and slowly, and stretch and massage the affected muscle. Make sure the person is not dehydrated.

stitch

A stitch is a common form of cramp that affects the muscles of th side of the body. It is usually associated with strenuous exercise.

how to recognize a stitch

The signs of a stitch are:

- cramp-like pains in the muscles in the side of the trunk
- history of recent exertion.

ction to take

low the exercise pace, and advise the person to breathe slowly nd deeply. If the pain is not relieved in a few minutes, suspect ne possibility of angina or a heart attack and seek medical help.

igh-risk sporting activities

ncreasingly, high-risk sports are part of the backpacking xperience. They include activities such as bungee jumping, vhite-water rafting, abseiling, parascending and gorge walking. he potential for injury with these activities is high, and probably ne most serious are head and spine injuries.

ead injuries

ll head injuries are potentially serious because there may also e damage to the brain. A head injury may lead to concussion – transient loss of consciousness followed by complete recovery a short time – and also to compression of the brain, which is fe threatening. It is therefore crucial to watch for a deteriorating evel of consciousness in anyone who has suffered a head injury.

oncussion

oncussion can also be thought of as 'brain shaking' inside the kull. It leads to a temporary disturbance of normal brain activity.

how to recognize concussion

The signs of concussion are:

- a brief period of impaired consciousness after a blow to the heac
- mild headache
- dizziness
- loss of memory.

action to take

Ensure that the person recovers fully and watch for changes in levels of consciousness or for strange behaviour. Get medical help if consciousness becomes impaired again or you are worried by the person's behaviour.

compression

Compression occurs when there is a build-up of pressure insid the skull as a result of bleeding inside the skull, or the brain itse swelling. It is a very serious and life-threatening problem that needs urgent medical attention.

how to recognize compression

The signs of compression are:

- recent head injury
- deteriorating level of consciousness
- intense headache
- noticeable change in behaviour such as irritability or disorientation

- noisy, slow breathing
- flushed face
- slow, strong pulse.

action to take

Get medical help as soon as possible. If the person becomes unconscious, place him in the recovery position.

key skills

If you suspect a person has suffered a head injury, check if he has lost consciousness. Observe any changes in consciousness or any abnormal behaviour. Seek medical advice.

5 • 5

spinal injuries

It is important to be aware of the possibility of an injury to the spine when a person has been thrown some distance. For example:

- fallen out of a moving vehicle or from a horse
- fallen from a height
- fallen awkwardly
- suffered a head injury
- dived into shallow water and hit his head.

how to recognize a spinal injury

You will recognize a spinal injury:

- from the type of incident
- by pain in the neck or back
- from the limbs feeling heavy or tingling
- by the loss of feeling in the limbs
- by loss of movement in the limbs.

action to take

Advise the injured person to lie still and ask for someone to help you. Get emergency help as soon as possible and do not move the person unless it is absolutely necessary. Steady and support the person by placing rolled up clothes around his head and neck, holding the head as still as possible. If the person is unconscious, open his airway using the jaw-thrust method.

how to do a jaw thrust

To use the jaw-thrust technique, kneel at the top of the person's head. Place your hands on either side of his face and put your fingertips behind the angles of his lower jaw. Gently lift his jaw forwards without tilting his head back.

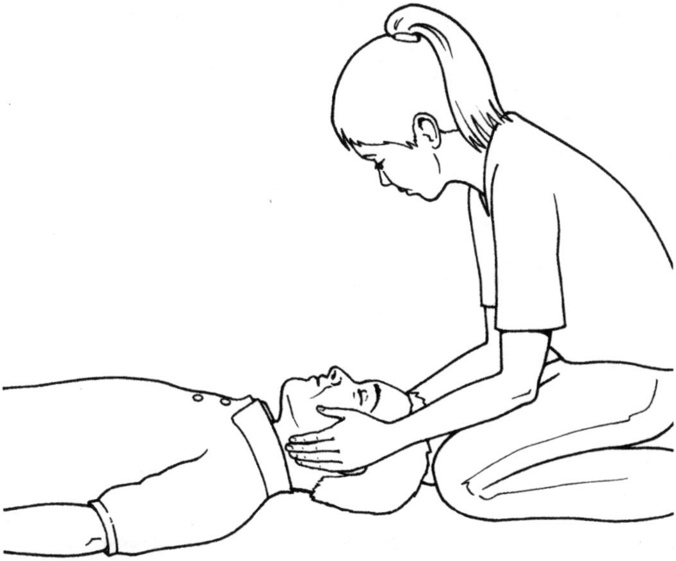

Fig 8 The jaw-thrust technique

one-minute wonder

Q If I can't maintain a person's airway by doing a jaw thrust, should I tilt the head back and turn him to the recovery position?

A The maintenance of an open clear airway has to take priority and so you should take all possible measures to try to make sure this happens and if that means turning the person into the recovery position, then yes. Try to get help to do this whilst still supporting the head and keeping the back as straight as possible.

summary

Conditions like diarrhoea, nausea and blistering can initially be an irritation and cause minor inconveniences. However, if they are left untreated these conditions can have more serious consequences.

Outdoor and sporting activities can be exciting and recreational. Make sure you take appropriate precautions and do not take unacceptable risks or participate in physically demanding activities while under the influence of alcohol or drugs.

self-testers

1 The signs of dehydration include:

- **a** feeling thirsty
- **b** having lots of energy
- **c** passing light-coloured urine
- **d** having muscle cramps
- **e** feeling dizzy

2 The treatment of diarrhoea includes:

- **a** having a long, cold drink
- **b** having frequent sips of cool water
- **c** eating a good meal
- **d** having no food until the appetite returns
- **e** having an alcoholic drink

3 Symptoms of altitude sickness include:

a nausea
b headache
c dizziness
d confusion
e inability to sleep

4 How would you treat a small cut on the leg?

a rinse the cut in cool water
b leave the cut moist
c apply a dressing
d change the dressing daily
e leave the cut open to the air

5 What are the common features of a blister?

a friction spot from a sock or boot
b pain when walking
c a prickly red rash
d a large bruise
e a sac of fluid

6 The signs of compression of the brain include:

a deep, fast breathing
b dry, pale skin
c mild headache
d disorientation
e flushed face

answers

1 **a**, **d** and **e**

2 **b** and **d**

3 **a**, **b**, **c**, **d** and **e**

4 **a** and **c**

5 **a**, **b** and **e**

6 **d** and **e**

7

camping and caravanning

Camping and caravanning are physically hard activities because they require putting up a tent or pitching a caravan, carrying water and making up beds. Associated activities like hiking and walking also increase the risk of injuries involving muscles, joints and ligaments. The potential for suffering a sprained joint, a strained muscle, a dislocated joint, or even a broken bone is high. In addition, because this type of activity is based on outdoor living, the use of campfires and barbecues heightens the risk of burns.

muscle strains

A strain occurs when a muscle is overstretched or partially torn. Any muscle may be affected, but those in the back, arms and legs are the most likely to be affected in camping and caravanning activities.

back strain

The most common cause of back pain is the overstretching of the back muscles. However, it is important to distinguish this from something more serious such as a disc problem.

how to recognize a muscle problem

The signs of a strained muscle are:

- dull, aching pain in the back
- pain that is worse when moving
- tightness of the muscles
- tenderness in the muscles.

action to take

If a person has strained his back, advise him to lie down flat until the pain eases. Painkillers can be taken. Encourage the person to resume normal activities as soon as the pain eases.

one-minute wonder

Q If the pain doesn't ease after a few hours, what should I do?

A This may indicate a more serious problem and so you should seek medical advice.

other muscle strains

Other muscle strains in the arms and legs have the same symptoms and should be treated using the RICE procedure:

Rest the injured site
Ice – apply a cold compress or ice pack
Compress – apply a firm roller bandage to compress
Elevate the injured limb.

how to apply a cold compress or ice pack to an injury

Partly fill a plastic bag with small ice cubes or use a bag of frozen peas. Wrap the bag in a dry cloth and hold it on the injury for ten minutes, replacing the pack as needed. Do not apply the pack directly to the skin, as it will lead to a cold burn. After cooling, apply comfortable, even compression to the injury site and surrounding the area with a thick layer of padding and securing the padding with a roller bandage.

how to apply a roller bandage

The rolled part of the bandage is called the head and the unrolled part the tail. Position yourself in front of the person on the injured side. Keep the injury well-supported while you are applying the bandage. Place the tail of the bandage below the injury and work from the inside of the limb outwards. Make two straight turns to anchor the tail in place. Then make a spiral of turns and work up the limb. Finish with one straight turn and secure the bandage with a safety pin or tuck in the end of the bandage.

After applying the bandage it is important to make sure it is not too tight and doesn't 'cut off' the circulation. Always ask if the bandage is too tight, and check the circulation below the bandage. Do this by briefly pressing a nail of the limb you are bandaging so that the nail blanches, and then release the pressure. If the colour does not return or returns slowly, the bandage is too tight and must be loosened and reapplied.

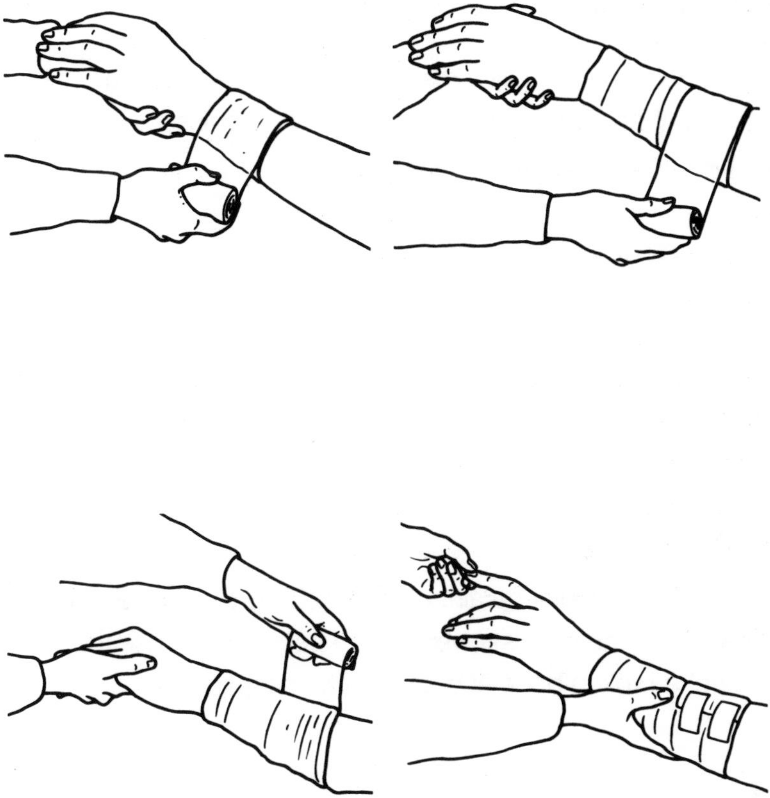

Fig 9 Applying a roller bandage

joint sprains

Joint sprains are usually a result of a sudden wrenching movement of a joint which pulls and tears the tissues around the joint, including the ligaments.

how to recognize a sprain

The signs of a sprain are:

- pain around the joint
- swelling around the joint
- tenderness and bruising at the site of the injury.

action to take

If you suspect a joint sprain, use the RICE procedure and take painkillers. If the pain is severe or the person can't use the joint, suspect a broken bone and arrange for hospital referral.

key skills

To treat a sprain or a strain, you should remember RICE: Rest, Ice, Compress and Elevate.

***one-minute** wonder*

Q What is the difference between a sprain and a strain?

A A sprain is a result of overstretching the supporting ligaments around a joint. A strain is a pulled or torn muscle.

***one-minute** wonder*

Q If I am walking in the hills and my companion falls and sprains his ankle, should I try to help him off the hills?

A This depends on the circumstances. Usually if a person has sprained his ankle he will be able to walk, but if the injury is more serious he will not. If he can't walk at all, you will have to call for help. If there is a risk of hypothermia, you must weigh up the pros and cons of staying or going. In this case, leaving the hill is likely to be the priority, so you should put on a supporting bandage and help him off the hill.

5 • 5

dislocations

A dislocation is a joint injury in which bones are partially or fully pulled out of their normal position. It is common in the shoulder, fingers and thumbs.

how to recognize a dislocation

The signs of a dislocation are:

- deformity at the joint
- difficulty with movement
- pain.

action to take

Advise the person to keep the joint still and support the joint in a position of greatest comfort. If the dislocation affects the shoulder or hand, immobilize in a sling and arrange for the person to go to hospital.

one-minute wonder

Q If I think a finger is dislocated can I pull it back into place?

A It is best not to try this as there may be a fracture accompanying the dislocation and you may do more damage. Also, pulling a dislocated joint is very painful.

how to improvise a sling

There are several ways to improvise a sling:

- use a jacket or cardigan corner – undo the jacket while the person is wearing it, fold the lower edge up over the arm and pin the hem corner to the jacket with a large safety pin.

- use a button-up jacket – undo one button while the person is wearing the jacket and place the hand of the injured arm inside the jacket
- use a long-sleeved shirt – lay the injured arm across the chest while the person is wearing the shirt and pin the cuff to the shirt.
- use a belt or scarf – make a large loop and put it over the person's head and then make a small loop and put the hand in it.

fractures – broken bones

When camping and caravanning, the most likely fractures are of the limbs, in particular the lower legs, and the arms.

facts about fractures

A fracture is a break in a bone. A fracture is described as 'closed' when the skin around it is intact. It is described as 'open' if there is an accompanying wound or the broken bone end is protruding through the skin. A fracture is described as stable when the broken bone ends do not move, either because they are not completely broken or because they are impacted, and it is described as unstable when the bone ends can move around. They can then damage surrounding tissues such as blood vessels and nerves.

how to recognize a fracture

The signs of a fracture are:

- pain
- swelling and bruising
- difficulty with moving
- deformity of the limb
- possibly a wound with the bone ends protruding
- signs of clinical shock (see Chapters 1 and 2).

action to take

If a person has a fracture, immobilize the fractured bone by holding still the joints above and below the fracture. If the bone ends are protruding through the skin, lightly cover them with a clean cloth, handkerchief or sterile dressing. Arrange to make the person comfortable for transfer to hospital. If emergency help is readily available, support and immobilize the broken bone by placing your hands above and below the fracture. To move the person some distance, get help to splint the broken bone and carry the person to where help is available. You can splint the bone by tying it to an unaffected part of the body, a walking pole or a piece of wood.

one-minute wonder

Q Is it true that a sprain is more painful than a fracture?

A It can be, but both injuries can be very painful and we suggest you do not use the amount of pain a person is experiencing to determine whether the injury is a sprain or a fracture.

crush injuries

Crush injuries usually result from dropping something heavy on to the foot or trapping fingers. They are often accompanied by broken bones and bleeding.

action to take

Release the person as quickly as possible. Stop the bleeding and cover any wounds. Support any suspected broken bones, and treat the person for clinical shock. Arrange for the person to go to hospital.

burns

The use of barbecues and campfires increases the risk of burns and scalds, and it is important to know how to treat them. We refer to burns as an injury resulting from contact with something hot or flames. Scalds are injuries that result from contact with fluids or steam.

how to recognize burns

Burns can be superficial, partial thickness or full thickness. A superficial burn involves only the outer layer of the skin.

A partial thickness burn involves the outer layer of the skin but includes blistering. A full thickness burn involves all the layers of the skin, and there may be damage to nerves and blood vessels. In full thickness burns, damage to the nerves can lead to a loss of pain sensation, and the skin looks waxy, pale and charred.

action to take

In the management of a burn, it is good practice to cool the burn to stop further burning (this can take up to ten minutes), and relieve the pain. First, remove any rings, watches or other constricting items before the swelling starts. Then, place the burn under cold running water or use a cold drink if water is not available. Do not use ice as this may cause a cold burn. After cooling, cover the burn to prevent infection. You can use a clean plastic bag, kitchen film, a pillowcase or a dressing to do this. If there is smoke, look for problems with the airway and deal with them (see Chapter 1, page 11). Treat any accompanying injuries. Access hospital treatment for all burns except those that are very small and not blistered.

things you should not do

You should not remove any clothing which is sticking to a burn, or apply sticky tape to the area around the burn because you can pull off more skin. Do not touch a burn or burst any blisters because this may lead to infection. Do not put on any lotions, creams or old-fashioned remedies as these can lead to infection. Do not overcool the burn as you may cause hypothermia.

key skills

To treat a burn or scald, place the affected area under cold running water for at least ten minutes. Cover with a clean pillowcase or dressing. Seek hospital treatment for all but the smallest of burns.

embedded fish hook

Fishing is often part of camping and caravanning, and if the barb of a fish hook becomes embedded in the skin it can be very difficult to remove. It is advisable to have the hook removed by a health-care professional but, if you are a long way from a hospital, this may not be possible and you might have to remove it yourself.

action to take

To remove a fish hook:

- if the barb is visible, cut it off and withdraw the hook by its eye
- if the barb is not visible, push the hook further into the skin until the barb emerges, then cut it off and withdraw the hook by its eye
- clean the wound and apply a dressing
- make sure the person is immunized against tetanus.

summary

Sprains, strains, burns and scalds are some of the more common injuries associated with outdoor activities such as camping and caravanning. Unfortunately, some people mistreat these injuries, and it is crucial to know the correct procedures. To treat a sprain or strain follow the RICE advice.

Burns and scalds are very painful. Your aim is to cool the area as quickly as possible to stop the cooking effect continuing. Do not use ice as this may cause a cold burn. Do not put ointment or cream on the burn as part of the initial treatment.

self-testers

1 Best practice when dealing with an ankle sprain is to:

- **a** elevate the leg
- **b** put on a cold compress
- **c** keep the ankle warm
- **d** encourage the person to walk
- **e** put on a firm bandage

2 When applying a cold compress to a muscle strain you should:

a apply it directly on to the skin
b use a bag of frozen peas
c keep it on for two minutes
d wrap it in a wet cloth
e replace the compress when it warms up

3 A fracture is:

a a broken bone
b open when there is an accompanying wound
c open when the bone ends stick out through the skin
d stable when the bone ends are impacted
e stable when the bone ends can move around

4 Best practice when managing a fracture of the lower leg is to:

a move the bone around to make sure it is broken
b cover any wounds or bone ends
c hold and steady the bone above and below the break
d use a walking pole as a splint
e move the person before putting on a splint

5 The management of a partial thickness burn to the hand includes:

a cooling it
b covering it
c popping the blister
d applying a moisturizer
e removing rings

6 When dealing with a superficial burn what should you avoid doing?

a applying lotions or creams

b cooling it under running water

c removing adherent clothing

d touching it with your fingers

e covering it with kitchen film

answers

1 **a**, **b** and **e**

2 **b** and **e**

3 **a**, **b**, **c** and **d**

4 **b**, **c** and **d**

5 **a**, **b** and **e**

6 **a**, **c** and **d**

8

travel health

Each country and region can present a particular risk of infection. In this chapter, we have identified some of the more common diseases, how they can be recognized and the actions you can take to remedy the conditions. Travelling around the world will always bring some risk to health but this can be minimized by taking some simple measures before setting out, including having the advised vaccinations.

planning ahead

By planning well ahead when you travel, many problems can be avoided.

action to take

Consult your travel health clinic or your own doctor at least two months before setting out. This will ensure that you have the necessary immunizations for the parts of the world you are travelling to and through. Even if you have to go at short notice, some preparation is better than none, so always ask for advice.

You will need to know where you are going, including any countries you may visit en route. You must also know if you are pregnant – this is especially important in the early stages of pregnancy as you may need to take precautions regarding what to eat and what medications to take. If you are planning to travel repeatedly, it is sensible to keep your immunizations up to date.

If you have not previously been immunized against diphtheria, polio or tetanus, before you travel is a good opportunity to have these. For all areas where standards of hygiene or sanitation may be less than ideal, hepatitis A and typhoid immunizations are recommended. For infected areas, anti-malarial pills and yellow fever are advised. In certain circumstances, meningitis, rabies, hepatitis B and tick borne encephalitis may be recommended.

Organize a basic first-aid kit, together with insect repellent and water purification tablets. Put together an emergency medical kit if you are going to a remote part of the world.

This should include:

- syringes
- five needles
- one dental needle
- one intravenous cannula
- one skin suture
- one packet of skin closures
- five alcohol swabs for skin cleansing
- one roll of tape
- dressings.

See page 147 for the recommended contents of a first-aid kit.

If you suffer from any ongoing illness, make sure that you take the necessary medicines with you. You may also need to take a letter from your doctor, or a personal health record card giving details of the drug/s prescribed in case you have problems with customs.

infectious diseases

hepatitis A

Hepatitis A is an infection of the liver, usually caught by consuming contaminated food or water. The virus is present in faeces so it can be passed from one person to another. Taking care with hand washing after going to the toilet and care over what you eat and drink are the best ways of avoiding the infection. There is a vaccine against hepatitis A. The infection is recognized from a general illness with fever, abdominal pain and jaundice (yellow pigmentation of the skin seen best in the white part of the eye). Because the illness involves the liver, paracetamol must not be given to relieve any fever because this may cause more damage.

hepatitis B and C

These are viral illnesses that occur worldwide and cause serious liver problems.

how to recognize hepatitis B or C infections

There may be no immediate signs of infection because these often appear after several weeks. The signs include:

- loss of appetite
- loss of weight
- abdominal pain
- nausea
- vomiting
- jaundice.

The infections are spread by:

- having unprotected sex
- sharing contaminated needles and syringes
- needle stick injury
- transfusions of contaminated blood
- use of poorly sterilized medical, dental, body piercing or tattooing equipment.

key skills

To help to avoid health problems while travelling find out about correct vaccinations to where you are going and make sure you have them.

one-minute wonder

Q What can I do to prevent hepatitis B infection?

A The best way to avoid infection is to avoid the high-risk activities listed on the previous page and to take a travel kit for use in emergencies. There is a vaccine available against hepatitis B that should be started six months before travel but there is no vaccine against hepatitis C.

HIV/AIDS

HIV/AIDS is a worldwide infection for which there is currently no vaccine. It is passed on in the same way as hepatitis B and C, and so avoiding high-risk activities (listed on the previous page) can usually prevent infection. It cannot be passed on through social contact, insect bites, poor hygiene or kissing, coughing or sneezing.

If you do have sex with a new partner always use a condom. Take condoms with you while travelling, as they may not be so available or such good quality in other countries. If you buy them in the UK, they should carry the British Standards kite mark or the European CE mark.

leptospirosis

This is also known as Weil's disease. Leptospirosis can be transmitted to humans who swim in water contaminated with the urine of many types of wild and domestic animals including rats. Warning notices are sometimes placed around potentially infected waterways. It can be a big problem for travellers who go swimming, canoeing, rafting or caving, and it is particularly a problem in the Caribbean and Hawaii. Covering all open wounds and not swallowing water can help prevent this condition.

how to recognize leptospirosis

The signs are:

- fever
- headache
- vomiting and diarrhoea
- marked redness around the eyes.

action to take

If you suspect leptospirosis, seek medical help as antibiotics will probably be needed.

malaria

Malaria is a parasitic disease spread through the bites of infected mosquitoes. Infection leads to fever and problems with the kidneys, liver, brain and blood, which can be fatal.

Malaria is present in all tropical climates, and some types are more virulent than others. It is advisable to take the appropriate anti-malarial tablets for the countries you are visiting. They must be taken as instructed, even if you are just passing through a malaria-infested area. You must keep on taking them for the recommended time after you return home.

one-minute wonder

Q What else can I do to try to prevent malaria?

A You can avoid mosquito bites by using insect repellent, keeping arms and legs covered, especially after sunset, sleeping in screened rooms, and using a mosquito net around the bed. Make sure the net has no holes, impregnate it with insecticide and make sure it is tucked in around the bed or mattress.

All these precautions do not, however, guarantee absolute protection. If you develop a fever or feel ill while abroad or up to three months after returning, seek medical help as soon as possible and always say where you have been.

key skills

Always seek medical advice if a person is unwell after returning from an area of the world where malaria is a problem.

rabies

Rabies is a serious viral infection transmitted by a bite from an infected dog, bat or other animal. The infection is characterized by headache, fever, fear of water, and seizures. It is usually fatal.

The virus can be found in the saliva of animals in Europe and North America as well as in less well-developed parts of the world. It is best not to touch any animals anywhere, even if they appear to be tame.

action to take

If someone is bitten by an animal, wash the wound immediately and vigorously with soap and water. Alcohol in the form of a cleansing wipe or alcohol spirit can be used to irrigate the wound. Get medical help without delay. Post-exposure treatment usually works provided it is administered quickly enough. Therefore, if you are bitten in a remote place and treatment is not available, contact the British Consulate's office (see page 157) to try to access the rabies vaccination.

Rabies immunization is recommended for backpackers and independent travellers undertaking long journeys in remote areas where medical treatment is not available. However, even if the person is immunized, this does not remove the need for urgent treatment if he is bitten by an infected animal.

ticks

Ticks are small parasites that live on sheep and deer, and carry a variety of diseases including lyme disease and tick borne encephalitis (TBE). They are present in the forested areas of Europe and North America including Austria and Scandinavia, and they are especially common in areas of thick undergrowth. Ticks are common in late spring and summer. They attach themselves to passing animals or humans and burrow into the skin, where they suck blood. When a tick is full of blood, it swells to the size of a pea and is easily seen. You must seek advice if you are going to thickly forested areas of Central and Eastern Europe because an immunization against TBE is available.

Lyme disease is characterized by:

- a skin rash usually on the upper arm, leg or trunk
- headache
- fever
- stiff neck
- muscle pains.

Treatment for Lyme disease is with antibiotics.

TBE is a serious problem that causes an inflammation of the brain.

To avoid being bitten when camping or walking in a tick-infested area, wear clothing that covers most of the skin, and use insect repellents. Inspect the skin regularly for ticks and, if you find one, smear it with vaseline if you have some and then pick the tick off with tweezers. If someone is bitten or starts to feel ill, seek medical help as soon as you can.

how to remove a tick

To remove a tick, grip the head of the tick close to the person's skin. Use tweezers if you have them. Use a to-and-fro action to lever the head of the tick out of the skin. Try to avoid breaking off the head and leaving it in the skin, as this will cause irritation.

yellow fever

The risk of contracting this dangerous virus is expected to rise. It is spread by mosquitoes in Africa and South America and, if a person gets the virus, he will suffer from headache, muscle pain, and a sudden high temperature. In severe cases it can lead to liver failure, kidney failure and death. Immunization is available and compulsory for visiting some countries.

one-minute wonder

Q Do I need to carry my certificate of immunization against yellow fever with me?

A Yes, many countries now ask to see a certificate of immunization in an attempt to keep the virus out of their country. Many countries will not allow you to even pass through without certification.

non-infectious problems

deep vein thrombosis

DVT (deep vein thrombosis) is a condition when a blood clot develops in the deep veins of the leg. It is potentially lethal if the clot moves around the body and settles in the lungs. DVT is increasingly associated with long-distance air travel but it is also possible whenever the legs are still for a long period of time. It may happen on car or train journeys. The risk is increased when pregnant or when taking certain medicines.

If a person develops pain in the leg either during or after travel, seek medical help as soon as possible.

one-minute wonder

Q What can you do to prevent DVT?

A If you think you are at risk, ask your doctor for advice before you travel. Consider wearing support stockings, keep moving and do exercises at regular intervals. Avoid dehydration by taking regular drinks, and avoid caffeine and alcohol.

jet lag

Jet lag is the result of travel across time zones, and will leave a person feeling tired and listless. It varies from one person to another but it is always best to avoid strenuous activity immediately after reaching a destination. Mental faculties will also be impaired so travellers should avoid signing complex contracts or agreeing to complex travel plans. Jet lag will take a few days to recede but sufferers will gradually feel better.

A few strategies may help:

- timed exposure to bright light
- altering clocks to the destination time and trying to think in that time
- careful use of sleeping tablets
- melatonin (a synthetic hormone that regulates sleep rhythms).

If a person is badly affected by jet lag, he should talk it over with a doctor to see if any of the strategies listed above can help.

summary

Avoiding some of the more common diseases is based on ensuring that vaccinations and immunizations are up to date. High-risk activities should be avoided, and ensure that you always have a medical and first-aid kit with you.

self-testers

1 Actions you should take before travelling include:

a have the necessary vaccinations for where you are going
b do not take medicines as they will be available where you are going
c put together a first-aid kit
d leave in a hurry without vaccinations
e take water purification tablets

2 If bitten by a dog in a remote area of the world, what should you do?

a ignore it
b wash the wound well
c check your anti-tetanus status
d mention it to your doctor on your return
e contact the British Consular office if anti-rabies vaccine is not available where you are

3 Hepatitis B and C and HIV/AIDS can be spread by:

a having unprotected sex
b sharing a used needle
c kissing
d body piercing
e tattooing

4 What are ticks?

a small parasites
b they are present on sheep and deer
c they are common in late spring and summer
d they are common in forested areas of Europe
e they are capable of causing Lyme disease

5 To try to prevent a DVT on a journey, what should you do?

a sleep for the whole journey
b drink lots of alcohol
c drink lots of water
d move around at regular intervals
e wear support stockings

6 To prevent malaria, what should you do?

a take anti-malarial pills
b use insect repellent in the morning
c keep arms and legs covered
d sleep under a mosquito net
e report to your doctor if you feel ill on your return

answers

1 **a**, **c** and **e**
2 **b**, **c** and **e**
3 **a**, **b**, **d** and **e**
4 **a**, **b**, **c**, **d** and **e**
5 **c**, **d** and **e**
6 **a**, **b**, **c**, **d** and **e**

9

medical emergencies

Medical emergencies can occur at home and abroad. However, when travelling abroad and participating in unfamiliar activities in a foreign environment, the risk of being faced with the medical conditions outlined in this chapter becomes more daunting.

Being exposed to new foods and insects may present a greater risk of an allergic reaction. In extreme cases, this could lead to anaphylactic shock. We have also covered the issue of choking. For many of us, choking can be an embarrassing incident that often occurs when we are in restaurants or public places but it is an incident that can be life threatening.

In this chapter we have tried to identify the more common conditions encountered whilst travelling.

choking

Because choking can develop into an emergency, it is important to take immediate action. Your aim when dealing with someone who is choking is to remove the object causing the problem. If the person is able to cough, encourage him to carry on. If he becomes weak or cannot cough anymore, bend him forwards and give him five sharp slaps between the shoulder blades. Stop if the object comes out or appears in the mouth. If back slaps fail, carry out abdominal thrusts (see opposite).

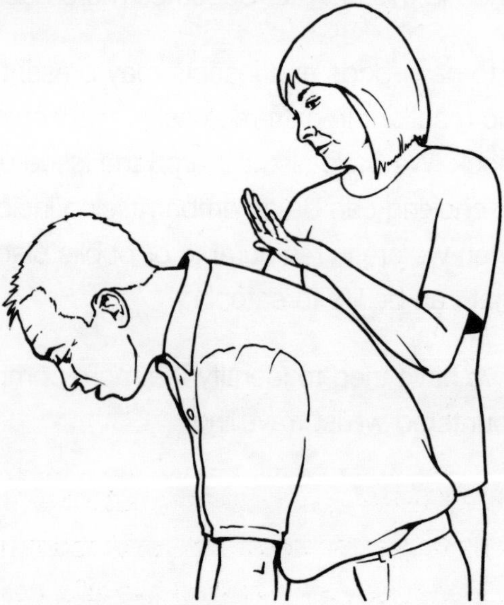

Fig 10 How to give back slaps to an adult

how to do abdominal thrusts on an adult

Stand behind the person and put both arms around the upper part of the abdomen between the navel and the bottom of the breastbone. Make a fist with your hands and pull sharply upwards and inwards five times. Check the mouth.

Fig 11 How to do abdominal thrusts on an adult

These measures will usually be successful but if they fail to remove the object, repeat the back slaps and abdominal thrusts three times and then check the mouth. If this fails, call for emergency help.

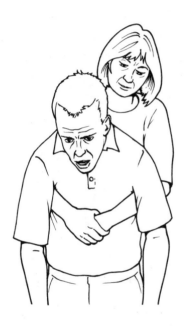

For a child between the ages of one and seven years old, the sequence is slightly different. If the child can cough, encourage him to continue. If he can't cough, give five back slaps. Check the mouth. If the back slaps fail, try chest thrusts (see below).

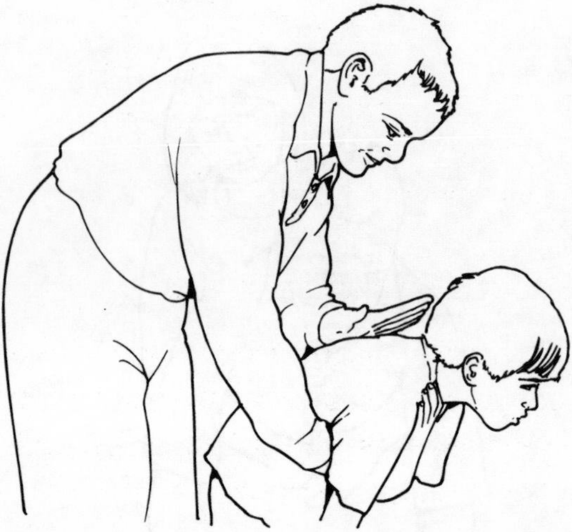

Fig 12 How to give back slaps to a child

how to do chest thrusts

Stand or kneel behind the child. Make a fist against the lower part of the breastbone and pull sharply inwards and upwards five times. Check the mouth. If this fails to remove the object, do five abdominal thrusts (see opposite).

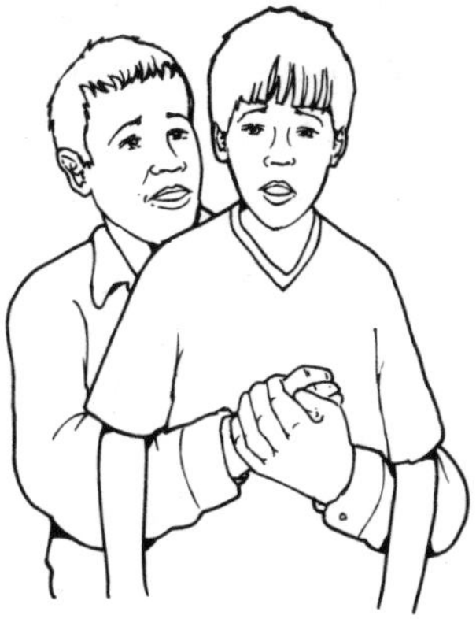

Fig 13 How to give chest thrusts to a child

how to do abdominal thrusts on a child

Stand or kneel behind the child and put both arms around the upper part of the abdomen between the navel and bottom of the breastbone. Make a fist and pull sharply upwards and inwards five times. Check the mouth.

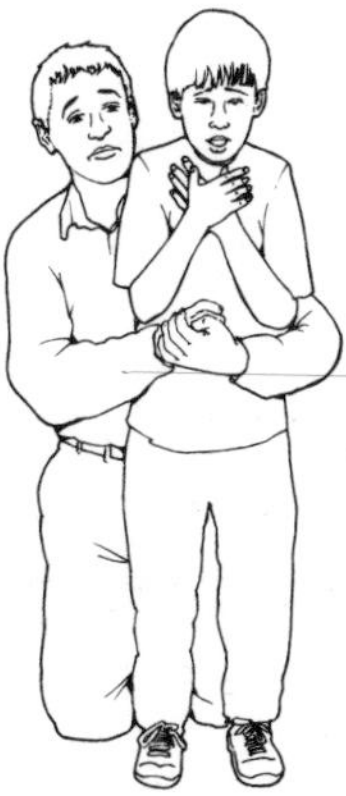

Fig 14 How to do abdominal thrusts on a child

If this fails, repeat the sequence of back slaps, chest thrusts and abdominal thrusts three times. If this fails, call for emergency help.

how to treat a choking baby

For a baby aged less than one year, the sequence is five back slaps and five chest thrusts using two fingers only. Do not do abdominal thrusts as they might damage internal abdominal organs.

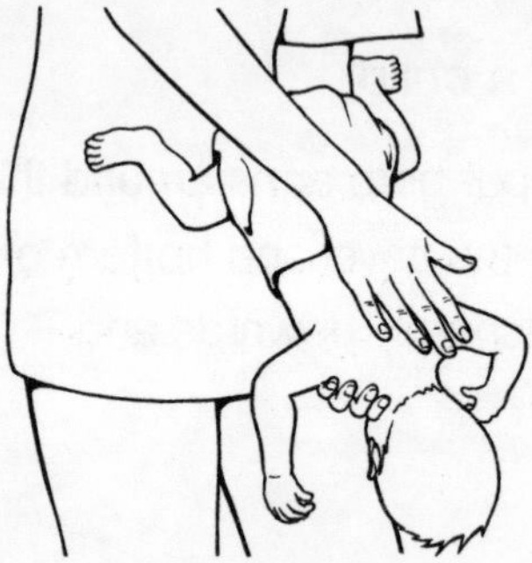

(a) How to give back slaps to a baby

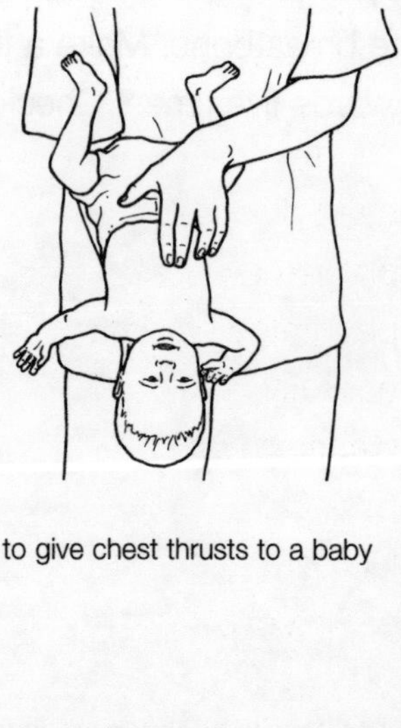

(b) How to give chest thrusts to a baby

Fig 15 How to treat a choking baby

At all times be prepared to carry out resuscitation as there is a risk that breathing will stop and consciousness will be lost.

***one-minute** wonder*

Q You say to give five back slaps. How hard should these be?

A They need to be sufficiently firm to cause a vibration in the chest to try and move the object.

diving accidents

Diving is a stressful sport. A depth change of 7 m produces changes in the body equal to a trip from sea level to the top of Mount Everest. There are many health reasons for not diving. These include:

- heart disease
- pregnancy
- perforated eardrum
- epilepsy
- diabetes
- migraine
- lung disease
- ear infection.

how to recognize diving complications

Complications of diving include:

- hypothermia (see Chapter 5)
- drowning
- marine bites or stings
- decompression sickness.

action to take

To prevent diving accidents, first of all make sure you are a good swimmer. Avoid dehydration, and do the deepest part of the dive first. Time the ascent, keep warm, and make a safety stop at 4.5 m. After the dive, move around to help nitrogen removal from the blood.

decompression sickness

Decompression sickness is an emergency requiring quick transfer to a recompression chamber. It usually results from ascending too quickly from a dive.

how to recognize decompression sickness

The signs of decompression sickness are:

- vomiting
- throbbing muscle pains
- mottled skin rash
- headache
- seizures.

drowning

Drowning is very common worldwide. When faced with a drowning incident, first follow the guidelines given in Chapter 1, page 8. The main problem with drowning is that fluid goes into the air passages and the lungs and stops the person from breathing. Any fluid causes irritation and narrowing of the airways initially, but later the irritation may lead to swelling of the airways and difficulty breathing. Therefore, anybody who is involved in a drowning incident must have a medical check.

action to take

If you are rescuing a person from water, once they are out of the water keep the head as low as possible to allow water to drain from the mouth, nose and upper airways. Keep the person warm – hypothermia is a potential problem if the person has been rescued from cold water. You will need to perform regular breathing checks (see Chapter 3). If the person is not responding, put him into the recovery position, monitor him closely and resuscitate him if necessary (see Chapter 3).

key skills

To treat a drowning victim, remove the person from the water and carry him with his head lower than his chest. Even if he appears to recover fully seek medical advice if you can. If he is not responsive, place him in the recovery position or resuscitate if necessary.

asthma

In an asthma attack, the air passages in the lungs narrow and breathing becomes difficult.

how to recognize asthma

- wheezing
- difficulty breathing, especially breathing out
- coughing
- distress and anxiety
- in a severe attack, inability to talk.

action to take

If a person has an asthma attack, try to keep calm, sit the person down and help him to locate and use his inhaler. A mild attack should ease in around three minutes. If it does not ease, use the inhaler again. If the inhaler has no effect after five minutes call for emergency help and be prepared to do resuscitation (see Chapter 3).

***one-minute** wonder*

Q If I have forgotten my inhaler, can I use someone else's?

A This is not a very hygienic thing to do, and you risk using the incorrect medicine for you. However, if the inhaler looks the same as yours and you are in an isolated location, then to use another person's medicine might be life saving.

5 • 5

insect stings

Insect stings are common when travelling, particularly if camping, hiking or backpacking. Stings are best avoided by using regular applications of strong insect repellent. In tropical climates, it is best to use a preparation containing Diethyl toluamide (DEET).

Normally an insect sting is more of a nuisance than a danger, but occasionally a person has an exaggerated allergic reaction to the sting and then an emergency situation arises. This is known as 'anaphylaxis' (see page 134).

how to recognize a sting

The signs of a sting are:

- pain
- redness and swelling around the site of the sting
- a visible sting.

action to take

If the sting is visible, scrape it off with your fingernail, credit card or the blunt edge of a knife. Do not use tweezers. Apply a cold compress. If the sting is on the hand or an arm, elevate the limb. If the sting is on the leg, firstly lay the person down and elevate it above the level of the heart. If the sting is in the mouth or throat, it can cause swelling and potentially block the air passages. Try to prevent swelling by putting cold water or an ice pack onto the sting. If the person who has been stung starts to have severe swelling, breathing difficulties or shock, call for emergency help as soon as you can.

key skills

To treat an insect sting if it is visible, scrape it off with a credit card or something similar. Apply a cold compress, and monitor the person for an abnormal reaction.

***one-minute** wonder*

Q Why can I not use tweezers to remove a sting?

A Because you will inject more of the poison into the person as you squeeze with the tweezers, and so risk the possibility of a severe allergic reaction to the sting.

5 ••••••••••••••••••••• 5

animal bites

If someone is bitten by an animal the wound is likely to be dirty. It may also be deep because an animal usually has sharp, pointed teeth. It is likely that antibiotics will be needed especially if bitten by a bat.

action to take

Wash the bite wound thoroughly with clean water and soap or detergent. Alcohol can be used to irrigate the wound. Dry the wound with gauze swabs or a clean cloth and cover the wound with a plaster if it is a small wound or a dressing if it is a large wound. If the wound is large it may need to be stitched, so medical help will be needed.

Make sure the person has been immunized against tetanus and if you don't, or are not able to, access medical help soon after the bite, make sure the wound stays clean. Consider the risk of rabies.

snake bites

There are many different types of venomous snake in different places in the world. The danger posed varies considerably, but the treatment of a bite is the same for all of them. To reassure you, not all bites inject venom and some inject only small amounts.

how to recognize a snake bite

The signs of a snake bite are:

- burning pain around the bite
- nausea and vomiting
- you should find out about the history of the incident – when it happened and what type of snake it was.

If the amount of injected venom is high, it can cause:

- dizziness
- fainting
- cold, clammy skin
- clinical shock.

action to take

If a person has been bitten the bite is usually on the lower part of the leg and the aim is to stop the spread of venom around the body. Help the person to lie down with his shoulders raised. Get emergency help. Gently wash the wound with cold water and roll on a light compression bandage above the bite. Immobilize the affected area if possible.

tetanus immunization

Hopefully the bitten person will be immunized against tetanus prior to travel. He should seek medical advice if he has never been immunized, if he is uncertain about whether or not he has been immunized and if it is more than ten years since the last injection.

stings and wounds from sea creatures

Jellyfish, Portuguese man-of-war, coral and sea anemones cause painful stings and some tropical sea creatures can cause severe poisoning.

action to take

To treat a sting, put on a cold compress to relieve the pain. If the sting is on a limb, raise the limb to reduce the swelling. If the sting is from a tropical jellyfish, pour vinegar or sea water over the injury to neutralize the sting. Then put on a light compression bandage above the sting and send for help. It is best to keep the person as still as possible until help arrives.

Spiny marine creatures such as sea urchins have spines that cause painful wounds in the feet when trodden on.

Immerse the feet in water – as hot as can be tolerated – for about 30 minutes. Do not bandage the wound, and have the spines removed in hospital if possible. If hospital treatment is not possible, remove the spines as carefully as you can.

anaphylaxis

Anaphylaxis is an exaggerated allergic response to a foreign substance in the body. The most common factors that precipitate a response are stings, venom, foodstuffs or drugs. These factors cause the release of chemicals into the bloodstream that narrow the airways and expands the blood vessels. The outcomes of this are a mixed picture of breathing difficulties and clinical shock, both of which are urgent problems.

how to recognize anaphylaxis

The signs of anaphylaxis are:

- anxiety
- red, itchy, blotchy skin
- rash
- swelling of the tongue and throat
- breathing difficulties
- wheezing and gasping for air
- signs of clinical shock (see Chapter 2, page 34).

action to take

If you suspect anaphylaxis, get help urgently. If the person is carrying an auto-injector, help him to use it. If there are breathing difficulties, help the person to sit up, but if there are signs of clinical shock, help the person to lie down and raise his legs. Be prepared to resuscitate (see Chapter 3).

key skills

Anaphylaxis is a serious condition, and if you think this is happening you need to act quickly. Check if the person has an auto-injector. If so, help him to use it. Be prepared to resuscitate.

summary

We have highlighted certain conditions in this chapter because they are among the most common things that happen and because in all of these situations there are some very practical things you can do to make the situation better. Early recognition of what is happening in many of the situations will make your first-aid response more effective.

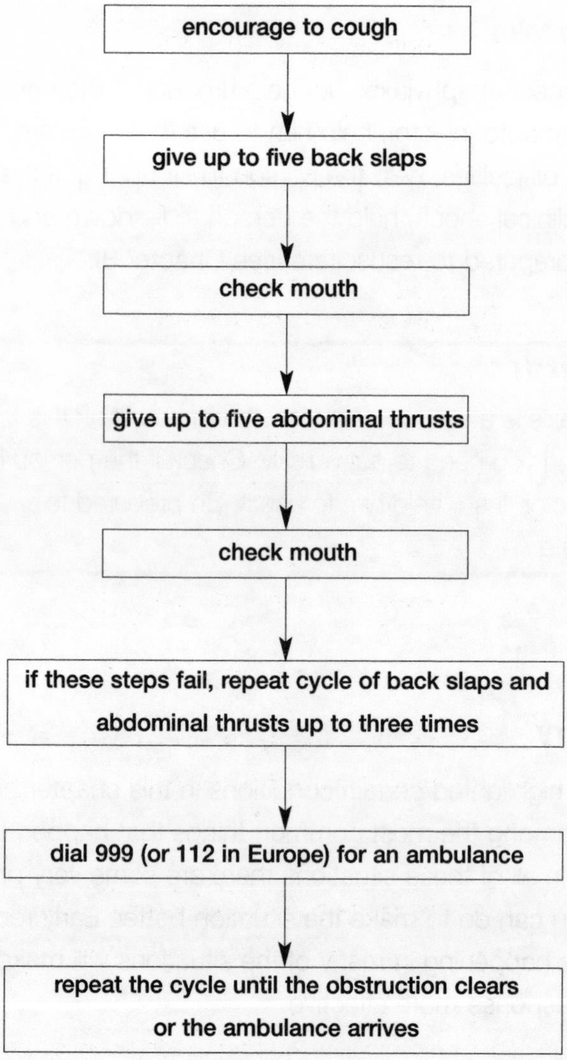

How to treat a choking adult

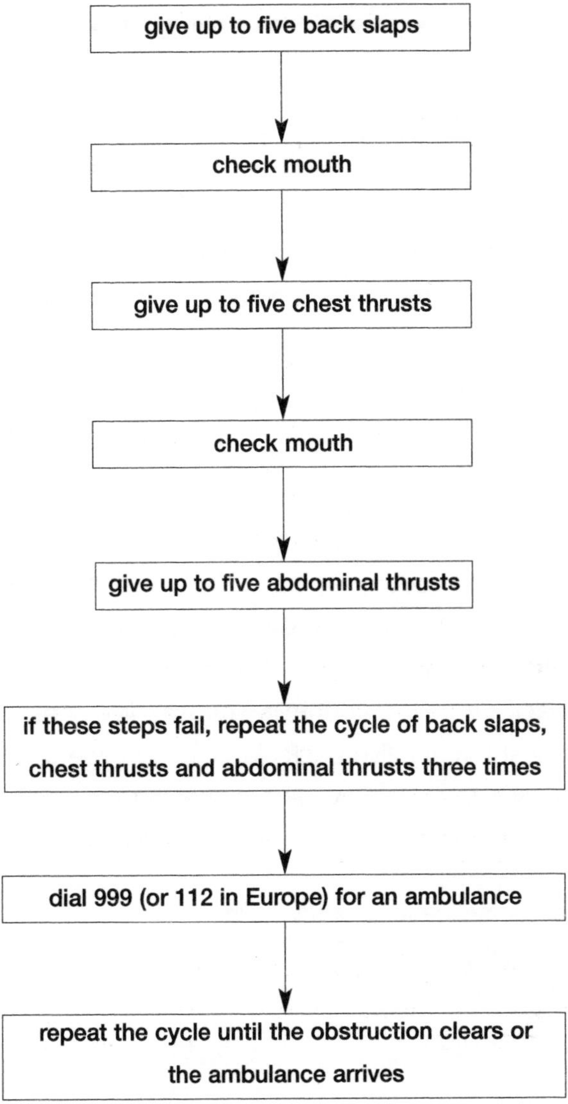

How to treat a choking child

self-testers

1 The sequence of actions for dealing with an adult who is choking is:

a encourage to cough, five chest thrusts, five abdominal thrusts

b encourage to cough, five back slaps. five abdominal thrusts

c five abdominal thrusts, encourage to cough, five chest thrusts

d five back slaps. five chest thrusts, five abdominal thrusts

e five abdominal thrusts, five chest thrusts, five back slaps

2 The sequence of actions for dealing with a child who is choking is:

a encourage to cough, five back slaps, five chest thrusts

b encourage to cough, give back slaps, five chest thrusts, five abdominal thrusts

c five back slaps, five abdominal thrusts, five chest thrusts

d five chest thrusts, five back slaps, encourage to cough

e encourage to cough, five abdominal thrusts, five back slaps

3 Common complications of diving include:

a jellyfish stings

b hypothermia

c heat exhaustion

d asthma

e decompression sickness

4 Symptoms of asthma include:

a wheezing
b coughing
c anxiety
d muscle cramps
e pins and needles

5 Insect stings are a problem because they cause:

a chest pain
b anaphylaxis
c skin redness and swelling
d pain
e throat swelling

6 What are the risks associated with a monkey bite?

a tetanus
b rabies
c Lyme disease
d malaria
e yellow fever

answers

1 **b**
2 **a**
3 **a**, **b** and **e**
4 **a**, **b** and **c**
5 **b**, **c**, **d** and **e**
6 **a** and **b**

case studies

Robert's story

Whilst walking in Turkey with a group of 12 people he hardly knew, Robert found himself in quite a sticky situation.

Walking deep in a valley, cut into the volcanic plateau of Capadoccia, the group were winding their way along a river path, which was poorly marked and full of brambles.

One of the group, a woman called Penny, was walking as she always did with walking poles, chatting to Robert about his work. Suddenly she decided to take a short leap across the stream; it was approximately 2 metres in width with a drop of half a metre from one bank to the other.

The crack was heard by the entire group – those that had already crossed the river turned, those still on the higher bank stared at Penny, now laying on the ground. Their faces drained of colour as they saw her foot now projected at a right angle to the side of her leg, floppy, still in its boot.

Everyone was paralysed for a few seconds until Penny's husband, David, and Robert knelt down beside her. She was ashen-faced and clearly in great pain. As David removed her boots, she hardly cried. 'A real tough cookie' thought Robert, which later proved to be the case.

'Go for help. Go for help!' David shouted to the guide, who was already trying to use his mobile phone to no avail – there was no signal at all. 'There won't be any,' replied Robert, but nobody could quite believe this until about ten minutes later when the guide returned, having run up the gorge side. 'There's nobody to help here. We have to get her to hospital ourselves,' he said.

Remembering everything he'd been taught on an aid workers' first-aid course, Robert had already planned the rescue but was careful to ensure that Penny was OK. There was no bleeding externally, no bone penetrating through the skin, but she was losing colour and her pulse was fairly rapid. Her husband wrapped her in more clothes while Robert, using a knife from his rucksack, cut down two small poplar saplings and trimmed the branches off. Three metres long and about 8 centimetres in diameter, these two trunks were to be a stretcher. 'Take off your shirts,' said Robert to the group. It wasn't what they had wanted to hear but they did as they were asked and each shirt in succession was threaded onto the stretcher poles (inside the shirt through the arms bunched up). Ten shirts were enough to form the stretcher. Then, with very little conversation but lots of co-ordination, Penny was lifted onto the make-shift stretcher, and a fleece carefully placed under her dangling foot.

Carrying a 50-kilogram woman for about a mile through undergrowth, across streams, and up unstable sandy arch slopes to the road was a tough challenge. The group formed a team, with one person supporting the foot, six carrying, two resting and two clearing a path at a time. Many had cuts and grazes which required attention later, but all managed the task and after about an hour and a half the group were able to get Penny to the road.

Eventually, after another 20 minutes, by loading her onto the back seat of a bus, the guide was able to get her to a local hospital along with her husband. However, they were unable to treat her so she was relayed, now on a drip, to a city hospital in a somewhat dilapidated ambulance. Two and half hours after the accident she was treated for a dislocated ankle and snapped fibia and tibia. Her bones were pinned and plated and after ten days she was flown back to the UK.

However, back at the roadside, whilst the guide and David accompanied Penny to the hospital on the bus, the temperature began to drop. The remaining ten people waited two hours for their mini bus to arrive from where it was supposed to meet them. In that two hours, to keep warm, they stuffed straw into their clothes and wore rucksack liners. Some were well kitted out, others weren't, the clothes were shared and they moved around to keep warm whilst waiting at a desolate pick-up point on the cold plateau. Robert and others cleaned up the cuts and grazed legs with clean water and issued neck scarves and tissues.

This situation had the markings of a real disaster but it worked out safely with the help of a little knowledge and a lot of luck.

authors' observations

This story highlights the importance of using whatever resources and materials are available.

Some might think this wasn't really first aid because nobody treated anybody but it really was exactly what first aid is all about – working together as a team, identifying the priorities of care using common sense and most importantly improvising. It also shows that these are situations when you have no choice other than to take the injured person to the ambulance rather than the more common scenario of the ambulance arriving at the person.

Barry's story

Barry George was enjoying his first family holiday in the sun with his grandchildren, it was the first time the whole family had been together for many years. In fact, it was the very first time he had been abroad with all seven grandchildren and their parents.

'A relaxing beach holiday was never my kind of thing,' said Barry. He preferred to be active and when the campsite nature warden asked for adults to volunteer to escort a group of children, including two of his grandchildren, on a 'mini beast march', Barry immediately volunteered. This 'march' involved a trek into the forest looking at and learning about the insects and wildlife that occupied the habitat.

The activities were always planned for early morning, when the temperature was lower and the chance of seeing more bugs and insects was increased.

'The warden was at the front of the group with me bringing up the rear, trying to keep the younger and more easily distracted children in front of me,' said Barry.

As they climbed a small hill, Barry began to feel a tightening of his chest and experienced some difficulty in breathing, this combined with a mild heartburn convinced him that the cooked breakfast he had eaten an hour earlier had given him indigestion. 'As the pain got worse, I called to the warden that I needed to sit down. When he came back to check up on me, the first thing he said was 'you're not looking too good.' By now Barry was feeling decidedly unwell, the pain in his chest was now working its way down his arms. It was at this point that Barry thought he was having a heart attack. The warden suspected the same and immediately radioed the campsite security telling them of their location and asking them to drive their off-road vehicle to the nearest point of contact. They were only a few hundred yards from the campsite, but Barry felt too unsteady to walk. While they were waiting for the vehicle to arrive the warden got the children involved in activities, aware that at least two of the children would be concerned for their grandad.

Barry was driven to the local clinic. 'The pain was so bad I never thought we'd get there' said Barry. They confirmed that the cause of the pain was a heart attack. He received a painkilling injection in the clinic and was then transferred to the hospital. It took two weeks to stabilize his condition and a further two weeks recuperation before he was well enough to fly home.

'I have never been so frightened in my life, all I can think of is if I had not gone with the kids I might have gone off on my own and I may not be here today' said Barry.

authors' observations

This reads like a textbook response to a potential life-threatening situation, the warden acted calmly and realized the need to get Barry to the clinic. We assume that because he knew the area well, he felt this was preferable to waiting for the emergency services to arrive (that is if they were able to get to Barry). It is not uncommon for some people to confuse a severe bout of indigestion with a heart attack. In this case the worsening chest pain radiating down the arms and the difficulty in breathing indicated something more serious. The warden did a very good job in reassuring Barry whilst also keeping the children occupied.

first-aid kit contents

There are no hard and fast rules about what should be in your personal first-aid kit. What you are most likely to need will depend on where you are and what you are doing. We recommend that you keep a fully stocked kit at home and in your car. However, for travel you may prefer to take a smaller, lighter kit for convenience.

There are some core items that we recommend you include in any kit:

- **plasters in assorted sizes** – these are applied to small cuts and grazes. Covering the wound with a clean, dry dressing will help prevent the area from becoming infected as well as help to stop any bleeding.
- **sterile wound dressings in assorted sizes** – these are used for wounds such as cuts or burns. Place the dressing pad over the injured area, making sure that the pad is larger than the wound. Then wrap the roller bandage around the limb to secure it.
- **triangular bandages** – commonly used for slings, these are strong supportive bandages. If they are sterile then they can also be used as dressings for wounds and burns.
- **safety pins** – useful for securing crêpe bandages and triangular bandages.

- **adhesive tape** – useful to hold and secure bandages comfortably in place. Some people are allergic to the adhesive, but hypoallergenic tape is available.
- **sterile gauze swabs** – these can be used to clean around a wound or in conjunction with other bandages and tape to help keep wounds clean and dry.
- **non-alcoholic cleansing wipes** – useful for cleaning cuts and grazes. They can also be used to clean your hands if water and soap are not available.
- **roller bandages** – used to give support to injured joints, to secure dressings in place, to maintain pressure on them, and to limit swelling.
- **disposable gloves** – these single-use gloves are an important safety measure to avoid infecting wounds as well as to protect you.
- **scissors** – using a round-ended pair of scissors will not cause injury and will make short work of cutting dressings or bandages to size. It is useful to have a strong pair that will cut through clothing.
- **insect repellent** – a protective spray against insect bites. Always follow the instructions provided. Never use repellents over cuts, wounds or irritated skin.
- **foil survival blanket** – this blanket provides protection from hypothermia caused by exposure to the elements and conserves body heat in cases of shock and trauma.
- **rehydration sachet** – to replace lost fluids and salts, dissolve a sachet in water and drink. This gives fast and effective replacement of body fluids during illness.

- **burn gel** – use directly on a burn to cool and relieve the pain of minor burns and to help prevent infection. Very useful if water is not available.
- **ice pack** – cooling an injury and the surrounding area can reduce swelling and pain. Always wrap an ice pack in a dry cloth and do not use it for more than ten minutes at one application.
- **tweezers** – useful for picking out splinters.
- **thermometer** – used to assess the body temperature. There are several different types including the traditional glass mercury thermometer and digital thermometer, as well as the forehead thermometer and the ear sensor. Normal body temperature is 37°C (98.6°F).
- **face shield or pocket mask** (a hygiene shield for giving rescue breaths) – these are plastic barriers with a reinforced hole to fit over the injured person's mouth. Use the shield to protect you and the injured person from infections when giving rescue breaths.
- **note pad and pen** – use the pad to record any information about the injured person that may be of use to the emergency services when they arrive. For example, the name and address of the person, how the accident occurred, and any observations. It is also useful to record vital signs so that you can monitor how well the person is doing over a period of time.
- **basic first-aid information** – a basic guide to first-aid tips, and emergency information (you can use the first aid essentials pull-out card in this book).

This is not an exhaustive list and there are many more items you may find useful to add to your kit. What is vital is that you have the necessary supplies ready to hand for when you need them.

Many people like to keep items such an antiseptic cream in their kits. The British Red Cross do not include anything which may no longer be sterile after the first use because of the risk of infection and allergies.

It is easy to make your own first-aid kit by collecting the items listed or, alternatively, you could simply buy a complete kit. For more information on British Red Cross kits, visit **www.redcross.org.uk/firstaidproducts** or call 0845 601 7105.

The Health and Safety Executive (HSE) is responsible for the regulation of almost all the risks to health and safety arising from work activity in Britain. Regulations concerning kit contents apply to employers. For more information about first-aid kits and training for the workplace, visit **www.redcrossfirstaidtraining.co.uk** or call 0870 170 9110.

household first-aid equipment

Throughout this book we have made reference to the importance of having first-aid skills, knowledge and equipment. In terms of equipment, we recommend you have a well-stocked first-aid kit (see page 147), but we also recognize that there are emergency situations where you will not have access to any of the equipment. In such situations you will have to be creative and use whatever equipment is available to you. In this section we have identified some of the items most of us already have in our homes and suggest how they can be useful in a first-aid situation.

- **beer** – you may not always have access to cold running water when treating a burn or scald. In this case, use some other cold liquid like beer, soft drink or milk. The aim is to cool the burnt area as quickly as possible using whatever cold liquid is available. Beer can be used to cool the area while waiting for water or while walking the person to a supply of cold running water. Remember, the area should be cooled for at least ten minutes for the treatment to be effective.
- **chair** – a chair has numerous first-aid uses; when treating a nosebleed, sit the person down while pinching the nose and tilting the head forward. If you are treating a bleed from a large wound to the leg, you should lay the person down and raise the leg above the level of the heart. A chair is ideal for this purpose.

- **chocolate** – chocolate can be given to a conscious person who is diabetic and having a hypoglycaemia attack known as a "hypo". This can help raise the person's blood sugar. Chocolate can also be given to a person with hypothermia as high-energy foods will help to warm the person up.
- **cling film** – cling film can be used to wrap around a burn or a scald once it has cooled. It is an ideal covering as it does not stick to the burn. It also keeps the burnt area clean and because it is transparent, you can continue to monitor the burn without removing the covering.
- **credit card** – when an insect sting is visible on the skin, a credit card can be used to scrape it away. Using the edge of the credit card, drag it across the skin. This will remove the sting. Using a credit card is preferable to using a pair of tweezers as some stings contain a sac of poison and if the sting is grasped with tweezers you may inject the sac of poison into the skin. If you do not have a credit card you can use the back of a kitchen knife or any other object similar to a credit card.
- **food bag** – a clean freezer or sandwich bag makes an ideal cover for a burn or scald to the hand. The injured part should be placed in the bag once the cooling has finished. By placing it in the bag you reduce the risk of infection and it also helps reduce the level of pain.
- **frozen peas** – frozen peas or other frozen small fruit and vegetables can be used to treat a sprain or strain. Wrap the peas in a tea towel or something similar and place them onto

the injury. This will help to reduce pain and swelling. Peas are ideal as they can be moulded around the injury more easily than bigger fruit and vegetables.

- **milk** – if an adult tooth is dislodged and cannot be placed back in its socket, it should be placed in a container of milk. This will stop it drying out and increase the possibility of it being successfully replanted by a dental surgeon.
- **paper bag** – a panic attack often results in the person hyperventilating (breathing very quickly). Reassure the person and get them to breath into a paper bag, this will help to regulate and slow down the persons breathing.
- **steam** – if your child has an attack of croup, sit your child on your knee in the bathroom. Run the tap to create a steamy atmosphere, this may help to relieve the symptoms.
- **vinegar** – if a person is stung by a tropical jellyfish, pour vinegar over the site of the sting. This will help to stop the poison spreading around the body.
- **water** – cold running water is the preferred treatment for burns and scalds. Place the burn under a cold water tap as quickly as possible and leave it there for at least ten minutes.
- **Yellow Pages and a broom** – in the event of having to provide assistance to a person with an electrical injury, where the person is attached to the current, you can stand on a copy of the Yellow Pages to insulate yourself from an electrical shock. You should then move the electrical cable away using a dry piece of wood, a broom handle is ideal.

about the Red Cross

the British Red Cross and the International Red Cross and Red Crescent Movement

The British Red Cross is a leading UK charity with 40,000 volunteers working in almost every community. We provide a range of high-quality services in local communities across the UK every day. We respond to emergencies, train first aiders, help vulnerable people regain their independence, and assist refugees and asylum seekers.

The British Red Cross is part of the International Red Cross and Red Crescent Movement, the world's largest independent humanitarian organization. This movement comprises three components: the International Committee of the Red Cross; the International Federation of Red Cross and Red Crescent Societies; and 181 National Red Cross and National Red Crescent Societies around the world.

As a member of the International Red Cross and Red Crescent Movement, the British Red Cross is committed to, and bound by, its Fundamental Principles:

- Humanity
- Impartiality
- Neutrality
- Independence
- Voluntary Service
- Unity
- Universality.

the International Committee of the Red Cross

Based in Geneva, Switzerland, the International Committee of the Red Cross (ICRC) is a private, independent humanitarian institution, whose role is defined as part of the Geneva Conventions. Serving as a neutral intermediary during international wars and civil conflicts, it provides protection and assistance for civilians, prisoners of war and the wounded, and provides a similar function during internal disturbances.

To find out more, visit **www.icrc.org**

the International Federation of Red Cross and Red Crescent Societies

Also based in Geneva, the Federation is a separately constituted body that co-ordinates international relief provided by National Societies for victims of natural disasters, and for refugees and displaced persons outside conflict zones. It also assists Red Cross and Red Crescent Societies with their own development, helping them to plan and implement disaster preparedness and development projects on behalf of vulnerable people in local communities.

To find out more visit **www.ifrc.org**

National Red Cross and National Red Crescent Societies

In most countries around the world, there exists a National Red Cross or Red Crescent Society. Each Society has a responsibility to help vulnerable people within its own borders, and to work in conjunction with the movement to protect and support those in crisis worldwide.

To find out more about the British Red Cross, visit **www.redcross.org.uk**

taking it further

useful addresses

Department of Health
www.dh.gov.uk/home/fs/en

Foreign & Commonwealth Office
King Charles Street London SW1A 2AH
www.fco.gov.uk

For up-to-date information on problems affecting your safety in around 200 countries refer to:
www.fco.gov.uk/countryadvice or contact:
Travel Advice Unit, Consular Directorate, Foreign & Commonwealth Office, Old Admiralty Building, London, SW1A 2PA
The telephone number for travel advice is 0870 606 0290
Fax: 020 7008 0155
E-mail: consular.fco@gtnet.gov.uk

NHS Direct
www.nhsdirect.nhs.uk
Tel: 0845 4647

The Hospital for Tropical Diseases

Mortimer Market Building, Capper Street, Tottenham Court Road, London, WC1E 6AU

Tel: 020 7387 9300 or 020 7387 4411

Fax: 020 7388 7645

www.thehtd.org/

This is an NHS hospital dedicated to the prevention, diagnosis and treatment of tropical diseases and travel-related infections.

International Red Cross contact details

Australia

National Office, 155 Pelham Street, 3053 Carlton VIC

Tel: switchboard (61) (3) 93451800

Fax: (61) (3) 93482513

E-mail: redcross@nat.redcross.org.au

www.redcross.org.au

Canada

170 Metcalfe Street, Suite 300 Ottawa, Ontario K2P 2P2

Tel: (1) (613) 7401900

Fax: (1) (613) 7401911

Telex: CANCROSS 05-33784

E-mail: cancross@redcross.ca

www.redcross.ca

Hong Kong
3 Harcourt Road, Wanchai, Hong Kong
Tel: (852) 28020021
E-mail: hcs@redcross.org.hk
www.redcross.org.hk

India
Red Cross, Building 1, Red Cross Road, 110001 New Delhi
Tel: (91) (112) 371 64 24
Fax: (91) (112) 371 74 54
E-mail: indcross@vsnl.com
www.indianredcross.org

Malaysia
JKR 32, Jalan Nipah, Off Jalan Ampang, 55000 Kuala Lumpur
Tel: (60) (3) 42578122/42578236/42578348/
42578159/42578227
Fax: (60) (3) 42533191
E-mail: mrcs@po.jaring.my
www.redcrescent.org.my

New Zealand
69 Molesworth Street, Thorndon, Wellington
Tel: (64) (4) 4723750
Fax: (64) (4) 4730315
E-mail: national@redcross.org.nz
www.redcross.org.nz

Singapore
Red Cross House, 15 Penang Lane, 238486 Singapore
Tel: (65) 6 3360269
Fax: (65) 6 3374360
E-mail: redcross@starhub.net.sg
www.redcross.org.sg

South Africa
1st Floor, Helen Bowden Building, Beach Road, Granger Bay, 8002 Cape Town
Tel: (27) (21) 4186640
Fax: (27) (21) 4186644
E-mail: sarcs@redcross.org.za
www.redcross.org.za

Taiwan and China
No: 8 Beixingiao Santiao, Dongcheng, East City District, 100007 Beijing
Tel: (86) (10) 8402 5890
Fax: (86) (10) 6406 0566/9928
E-mail: rcsc@chineseredcross.org.cn
www.redcross.org.cn

index